I0493648

CARING FOR SENIORS

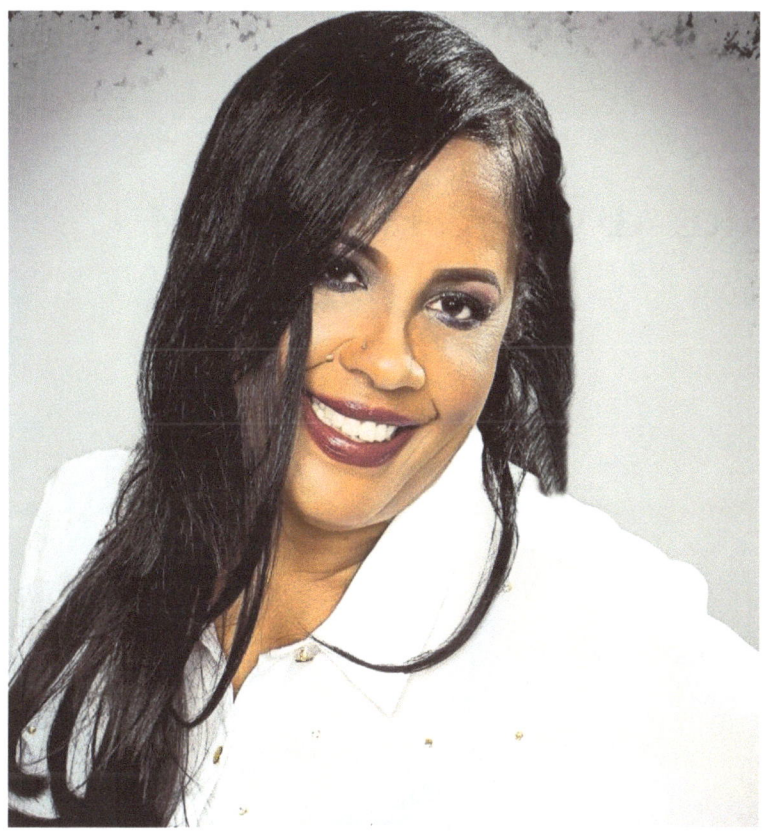

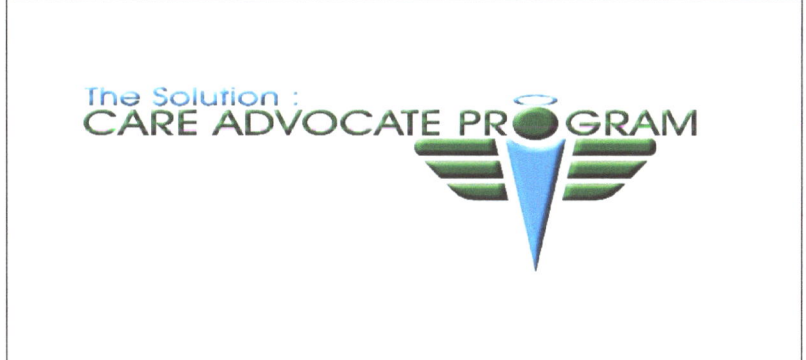

CARE ADVOCATE PROGRAM

Dr. Rita Elaine Stuckey

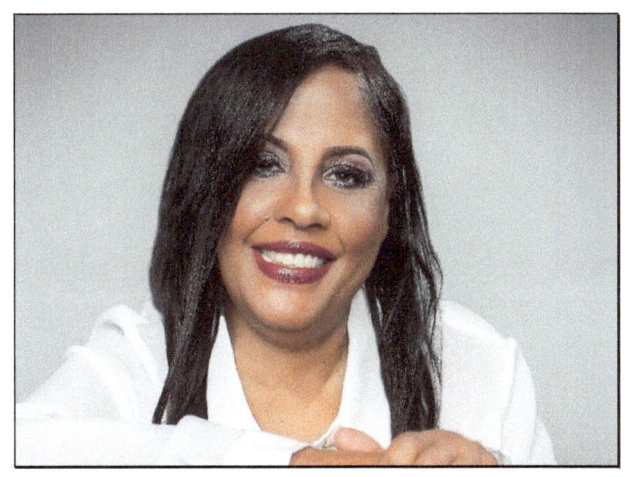

DR. RITA DEDICATED HER LIFE TO SENIORS, FAMILIES AND COMMUNITIES TO PROMOTE SAFE ENVIRONMENTS OF CARE FOR THE ELDERLY

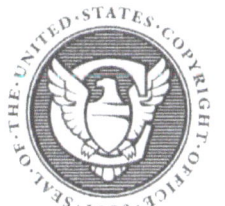

Certificate of Registration

This Certificate issued under the seal of the Copyright Office in accordance with title 17, *United States Code*, attests that registration has been made for the work identified below. The information on this certificate has been made a part of the Copyright Office records.

Maria A. Pallante

Register of Copyrights, United States of America

ABSTRACT

Question: As a result of a four month Care Advocate Program Training (C.A.P.): What will participants learn about elder abuse in institutional settings after completing the training program? Will participants be able to identify, intervene and report elder abuse if it is suspected? Will participants learn to advocate on behalf of residents and their families?

Relevance: A study was conducted by nine members of Congress to investigate the conditions of nursing homes in the San Francisco Bay Area. This study inspected 288 nursing homes that accept residents covered by Medicare and Medicaid programs serving approximately 22,000 residents. The investigation found that only 18 out of 288 nursing homes met full or substantial compliance with federal nursing home standards. In contrast, 119 nursing homes - more that one out of three- had violations that caused actual harm to residents or placed them at risk of death or serious bodily injury at the hands of paid caregivers employed by the facility.

Methods: The Care Advocate Program training was conducted at Allen Temple Baptist Church in Oakland. The C.A.P. trainees attended three consecutive Saturdays of four-hour classroom training and performed four facility site visits to an Allen Temple member residing in a nursing home. Trainees completed a sequence of questionnaires intended to gain insight into the effectiveness of C.A.P. program and used to evaluate areas of program improvement. The data collection tools included: a pre-test, facility checklist, observation checklist, and post-test and family communication form. A list of

Allen Temple members residing in an institutional setting is provided in the weekly church bulletin and was used to identify seniors who could participate in the C.A.P. program. Informed consents were obtained and trainees conducted unannounced facility visits.

Data: At the end of the four month Care Advocate Program training, an evaluation of the program was conducted to determine if participants were able to: 1) identify the signs and symptoms of elder abuse 2) intervene when abuse is suspected 3) report abuse to appropriate protective service agencies 4) advocate on behalf of the senior and their families.

Analysis: The data collection tools were used to determine whether trainees were able to identify the characteristics of abuse, what methods trainees took to intervene on behalf of the senior if abuse was recognized, what steps were taken to report elder abuse to protection and if trainees advocated on behalf of residents and their families in addressing abuse.

Implications: Findings of the evaluation study for the Care Advocate Program will prove useful in addressing elder abuse, develop training of volunteers to advocate and empower residents and their families, maximize effective elder abuse preventive measures and initiate broader public policy changes to ensure the safety of residents in institutional settings.

TABLE OF CONTENTS

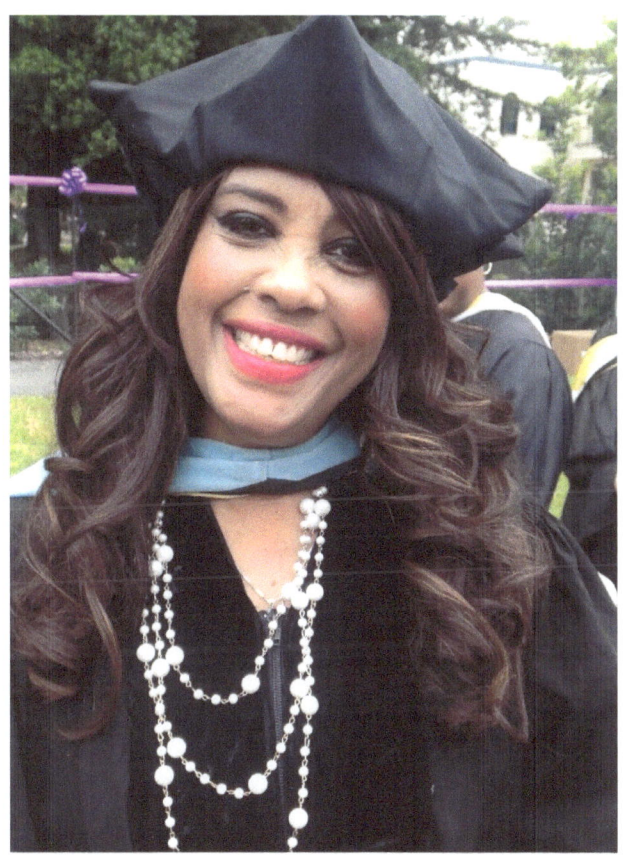

MILLS GRADUATE 2001 AND 2005

I am delighted that you are being recognized as a national leader in developing effective ways to curtail elder abuse in long-term care facilities. The Mills community is so proud of you and we applaud your many achievements. We are also please that you are such an outstanding role model for our students and that you have been a prominent member of the alumnae community as a mentor and a leader.

-Alecia A. DeCoudreaux, President Mills College

PREFACE

While contracting as the Interim Director of Nursing for a ninety-nine-bed nursing home in the Bay Area, I witnessed all levels of abuse against residents. The nursing staff were hitting, biting, spitting, stealing and sodomizing elderly residents. I was appalled at the incidents of abuse that residents were being subjected to when the owner, administrator and management team all had full knowledge of the situation. They stood by and did nothing.

I witnessed a male nurse repeatedly sodomizing elderly female residents, leaving semen on their face and clothing and openly bragging about how he had done it and whom he would do next. The medication nurse continuously pocketed patient medications and stole narcotics from locked cabinets for personal use and street sales. Nursing home staff engaged in thievery of patient belongings and prying gold out of resident's dentures for monetary gain, often taking bets as to who would get it first.

Bedsores went untreated by the wound care nurse who documented in the resident's medical record that treatment had been rendered, resulting in questionable resident deaths. The Director of Social Services solicited sexual favors from family and visitors in the parking lot as they left the facility. Management insufficiently rationed protective undergarments, paid for by the resident's family, forcing nursing staff to use bed linen as diapers. Numerous accounts of rats found chewing on resident's feeding tubes, their only source of nourishment, continually reported to supervisors by concerned nursing staff.

True-life stories regarding the harsh reality of elder abuse is commonplace and nursing homes are currently admitting registered sex offenders into these settings.

This situation upset me deeply and I called my father, Attorney Felix Stuckey, to inform him that I would be firing four nurses who had been abusing seniors in this facility for at least five years. I knew that my license and safety were in jeopardy and wanted my father to be aware of the situation in case any legal ramifications for "telling" of the abuse occurred. I drove to the Emeryville marina and cried to God to help me protect these and other vulnerable seniors from abuse.

The next day I received a telephone call from Professor Pete Mesa at Mills College asking that I meet with him to discuss my application to the doctoral program. It was imperative that I prepare myself academically to be a voice of advocacy for seniors residing in nursing homes and their families by completing a doctoral degree. These drastic senior abuse stories, challenging management experiences and deeply personal affects observing abuse had on my heart are what motivated me to write this book. Together we can ensure a safe environment of care for our seniors.

ACKNOWLEDGEMENTS

Allen Temple Baptist Church

Pastor Dr. J. Alfred Smith Sr.

Pastor Dr. Earl C. Stuckey

Pastor Dr. Gillette O. James

Laurinda Ochoa - District Attorney

Rhonda Theisen - District Attorney

Victoria Tolbert - Adult Protective Services

Ombudsman

Attorney Prescott Cole - C.A.N.H.R.

Sergeant David Faeth - Oakland Police Department

Dr. H. Geoffrey Watson - Internist

Dr. Kevin Smith- OB/GYN

Dr. Michael Hebrard- Physiatrist

Pamela Aziz - Nutritionist

The Stuckey Family

**Special acknowledgement
to all long-term care
facilities providing quality
care to seniors**

SPECIAL THANKS

Dr. J. Alfred Smith Jr.

Mills College

Dr. Joseph Kahne

Dr. Linda Perez

Dr. David Donahue

Professor Emeritus Pete Mesa

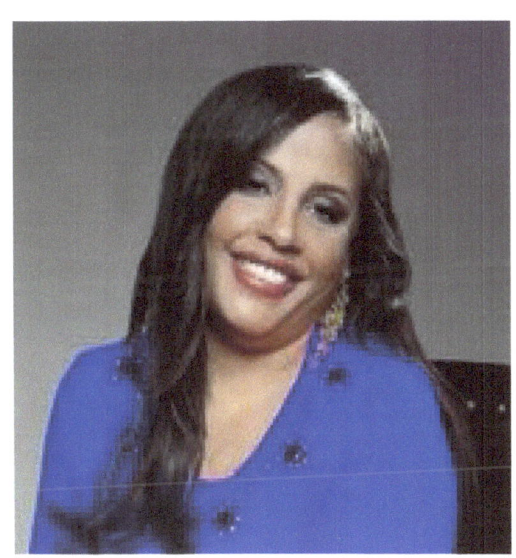

**Appreciation to the
participants of the
Care Advocate Program
whose names are protected to
ensure confidentiality**

I. Problem

Abuse violations are among the most serious violations that can occur in nursing homes. The elderly and disabled residents living in nursing homes cannot protect themselves from physical attack or sexual assault. Sometimes they cannot even communicate to family members that they have suffered abuse. Residents and their families are entirely dependent upon nursing homes to ensure the safety of residents (Waxman, 2001).

Consider for example the case of Helen Love, a 95-pound bedridden woman that resided at Valley Skilled Nursing in Sacramento, California. Nursing home abuse was reported by CBS news when a staff member attacked this 75-year old woman and left bruises to her neck, chin and legs. Around 7 p.m. on his eighth day on the job, certified nursing assistant Tim Saelee entered Love's room and found that she had soiled herself and needed cleaning. That upset Saelee so he began handling her roughly. According to Love and a witness, when she complained, Saelee attacked her, got ferocious and starting beating her all around the bed. *He dislocated her neck, broke her wrist and she was covered with bruises.* Love decided that the only way she could survive was to play dead which caused Saelee to eventually leave the room. Love's son wanted to take his mother to a hospital emergency room a block or so away but the nursing home refused to release her. Gary Love stated that it was only after he threatened to call the police that the administrators backed down.

Emergency room doctors quickly discovered that she had a dislocated neck and a broken wrist. Her condition was so grave that doctors were afraid to operate on her neck. Instead

2

they drilled holes in her skull and fitted her with a steel halo to hold her head up. It was a painful and draining treatment. According to the nursing home doctor's report, "There was no head injury, no loss of consciousness and x-rays did not disclose any fracture of the mandible, forearm or wrist. The nursing home doctor said any bruising Love had was caused by her "medical illness". When asked if she tried to fight back, Love said. "Oh, I'm not a quitter; I'm a fighter. I was going to fight and now I'm black and blue all over." This was not the first time Saelee was accused of abuse and had been warned about rough handling patients at another Sacramento nursing home. Then he was fired for threatening to hit a resident. He was hired one month later at Valley Nursing Home facility. At this facility three other employees had convictions for abuse, which under the state law should have prohibited them from working in a nursing home.

The nurse's assistant pleaded guilty to elder abuse and got one year in county jail. The California Department of Health Services told CBS NEWS that it has revoked the license of another nurse assistant employed at the Valley Nursing Home facility. This facility is the parent company to North American Healthcare that operates 17 facilities in California and has applied to open three more homes in California but was turned down by the state in September 1999 because of "consistently poor care" in their facilities. In this case and across the nation, dangerous nursing home workers are not being detected, and elderly people certainly are not being protected. At least 33 states do some kind of background check on a very small number of nursing home workers *but none require a national background checks.* A recent government report found that state background checks aren't working, saying, "There was no assurance that individuals who may pose a risk to residents are systematically identified and barred from nursing home employment." (CBS News, 2001).

Two days after the videotaped interview, Helen Love died.

CBS News reported the following statistics on Elder Abuse in Nursing Homes:

- The United States Census Bureau projects that California's elderly population will nearly double within the next 20 years - from 3.7 million to more than 6.4 million.

- The United States General Accounting Office claims that more than 43 percent of all Americans over the age of 65 will reside in a nursing home sometime in their lives.

- In 1998, the United States General Accounting Office reported that one in three California nursing homes was cited for serious or potentially life-threatening care problems.

- In 1999, the U.S. Congress Committee on Government Reform (USCCGR) reported that of the 439 nursing homes in Los Angeles County, only one was in total compliance with federal standards of care.

- In 2000, the USCCGR reported that only 18 of the 288 nursing homes in the San Francisco Bay Area were in full or substantial compliance with federal standards of care.

- In 2001, the USCCGR reported that all 27 of the nursing homes in the 22nd congressional District (Santa Barbara) violated federal health and safety standards.

Institutional elder abuse often goes undetected, unreported and unaddressed because of inadequate internal systems to detect abuse; neglect and mistreatment of the elderly inflicted on them by paid caregivers primarily employed nurses' aides (Waxman, 2001).

Common problems found in these settings include untreated bedsores, inadequate medical care, malnutrition, dehydration, preventable accidents, and inadequate sanitation and hygiene (Ruppe, 2001). Elderly people were abused in nearly a third of the nations' nursing homes in the past two years, many of them suffering serious injuries such as hip fractures. Henry Waxman, the top Democrat on the House of Government Reform Committee, states that an investigation on nursing homes found thousands upon thousands of incidents of unconscionable abuse against the elderly (USA Today, 2001).

The results of this investigation conducted by the Special Investigations Division of the U.S. House of Representatives, documented that numerous institutional settings fail to protect and do not intervene when staff members abuse residents (U.S. House of Representations, 2001). This report clearly revealed how State inspectors in many cases discovered that residents *did* report the abusive incident to nursing home staff and/or facility managers who neither investigated the allegations nor reported the allegations to proper authorities. Investigators said many violations are neither detected nor reported; leading officials to believe the problem is underestimated (USA Today, 2001). Data analysis also revealed that situational characteristics are the best predictors of patient maltreatment. Staff burnout and level of staff-patient conflict were both strongly related to abuse of patients (Pillemer& Bachman-Prehn, 1991).

All abuse is on the rise with more that than twice as many nursing homes being cited for abuse in 2000 than in 1996. In 1996, 5.9 percent of all nursing homes were cited for an abuse violation during their annual inspections; in 2000, 16 percent of nursing homes were cited (McQueen, 2001). Not only did patients suffer unnecessary deaths and injuries due to abuse and neglect, but also efforts by state and federal regulators to halt these catastrophic outcomes were often not effective (Grinfeld, 2000). A CBS News analysis of the federal government's nursing home inspection database finds more than 1,000 nursing homes were cited last year for hiring staff with a history of abuse. Federal regulators admit, however, that the statistics conceal how bad things really are inside America's nursing home. State inspections are often unreliable, and most problems in nursing homes go unreported. That's especially true when it comes to cases of physical abuse. The Love family knows all too well.

II. LITERATURE REVIEW

The Problem and the Growing Need for Nursing Home Care

Abuse and neglect of the elderly in institutional settings, primarily nursing homes, is increasingly recognized as a widespread national tragedy in the United States. Over thirty percent of the nursing homes in the United States- 5,283 nursing homes- were cited for an abuse violation that had the potential to cause harm between January 1999 and January 2001 (U.S. House of Representatives, 2001). These nursing homes were cited for almost 9,000 abuse violations in this two-year period. According to this recent report, *Abuse of Residents Is a Major Problem in U.S. Nursing Homes*, over 2,500 of the abuse violations were serious enough to cause actual harm to residents or to place residents in immediate jeopardy of death or seniors injury (U.S. House of Representatives, 2001).

Many families are becoming increasingly concerned about the conditions in nursing homes. The country is graying at a rapid rate—In 1966, there were 19 million Americans 65 years of age and older (Health Care Financing Administration, 1998). That figure has now risen to 34.6 million Americans, or 13% of the population (U.S. Census Bureau, 1999). In 25 years, the number of Americans aged 65 and older will increase to 62 million, nearly 20% of the population (U.S. Census Bureau, 1996).

This aging population will increase demands for nursing home and long-term care. There are currently 1.6 million people living in almost 17,000 nursing homes in the United States (Block, 1999). The Department of Health and Human Services (DHHS) has estimated that 43% of all 65 year olds will use a nursing home at some point during their lives (HCFA Report to Congress, 1998). Of those residents that need the services of a nursing home, more than half will require stays of over one year, and over 20% will be in a nursing home for more than five years. The total number of nursing home residents is expected to quadruple from the current 1.6 million to 6.6 million by 2050 (American Health Care Association, 1999).

Nursing Home Care is Big Business

The Health Care Financing Administration (HFCA, 1998) studied the economic dynamics surrounding the nursing home industry in a funding report. They found that private for-profit companies run most nursing homes. Of the 17,000 nursing homes in the United States, over 11,000 (65%) are operated by **for-profit** companies. The five largest nursing home chains in the United States operated over 2,000 facilities and had revenues of nearly $14 billion in 1998.

In 2000, it is projected that federal, state, and local governments will spend $58.1 million on nursing home care, of which $44.9 billion will come from Medicaid payments ($27.7 billion from the federal government and $17.2 billion from state governments) and $11.2 billion from federal and Medicare payments. Private expenditures for nursing home care are estimated to be $36 million ($29.2 billion from residents and their families, $5 billion from insurance policies, and $1.8 billion from other private funds (HFCA, 1998).

Due to the expected growth in nursing home residents, public awareness of violations of nursing home standards have increased interest and concern regarding recent annual inspections conducted by the California Department of Health and Human Services in 1999. The annual inspections cited many examples of routine violations of federal standards governing quality of care, violations that cause actual harm, neglect and mistreatment of nursing home residents (DHHS, 1999). The results indicate that many residents are not receiving the care that their families expect and that federal law requires. Examples of these violations are as follows:

- A resident was admitted to a nursing home with three pressure sores. Due to improper care, she developed five more sores, which became severely infected. When the resident was transferred to a hospital, her condition had deteriorated so much that her husband and physician decided that only care and comfort measures would be provided and that aggressive treatment of sores would not be pursued. She died ten days later (State Citation, 1999).

- A 73 –year- old resident was found slumped over in her wheelchair during mealtime by a nurse. The resident had stopped breathing. Rather than immediately performing CPR on the resident, the nurse wheeled her 100 yards down the hall and called 911. The resident suffered extensive brain damage and died (State Citation, 1999).

- One facility had orders to swab a stroke victim's mouth two to three times a day. However, the resident's son testified that whenever he visited his mother that she had a thick brownish substance in her mouth. The resident subsequently died from pneumonia due to aspiration of oral secretions (State Citation, 1999).

These findings are consistent with a spate of reports on institutional elder abuse that brought the issue to public awareness in the late 1970's early 1980's through research findings and Congressional hearings. A 93-volume, 74,000-page, federal report released May 1990 on 15,000 nursing homes across the USA and their 1.3 million patients (Senior-Site, 1990) concluded:

- 24% improperly administered drugs according to the written orders from the attending physician (60% in New Jersey):

- 26% did not provide adequate personal hygiene (67% in the state of Washington);

- 21% did not follow proper isolation techniques to prevent the spread of infection;

- 20% did not provide each resident with a urinary catheter with proper routine care;

- 36% did not follow rules requiring that food be stored, prepared, and served under sanitary conditions (62% in Alabama);

- 18% failed to provide patient's bathroom needs according to federal standards (33%in Michigan);

- 12% did not properly treat bedsores; and

- 15% did not provide patient with privacy during treatment and personal care.

Similarly, recent studies by the federal U.S. General Accounting Office (GAO) have indicated that many nursing homes fail to meet federal and safety standards (Thompson, 1998). The GAO also reports that even in cases where penalties were imposed on such facilities, improvements were often only temporary; many were again out of compliance by the time the next survey or follow-up inspection was conducted (ABC News, 2001).

Senator Charles Grassley (R-Iowa), the chairman for the Committee on Aging, found after an extensive study, *that one in three nursing homes is plagued by "seriously or potentially life-threatening problems" and that the same problems probably exist across the nation* (Freidman, 2000). The incidence of threatening problems in nursing homes led Time to report on a study last fall by Palo Alto, Calif., attorney Von Packard and investigators Robert Bauman and Dina Rasor of the death certificates of all Californians who died in nursing homes from 1986-1993. In more that 7% of the cases, lack of food or water, untreated bedsores or infections were listed as a cause of death (Thompson, 1998).

This probe led Senator Grassely to order the GAO to California to investigate. The GAO's medical review of 62 residents who died in trouble-prone California nursing homes showed that 34 of them received poor care that probably contributed to their demise. Applying the GAO's percentage of negligent California deaths to the nation's nursing- home population suggests that close to 20,000 U.S. nursing-home residents are *dying prematurely or in unnecessary pain, or both* (Thompson, 1998). The most alarming conclusion drawn by GAO is its belief that the extent of current serious care problems portrayed in these federal and state data is likely to be understated.

A report was prepared on July 30, 2001 at the request of Rep. Henry A. Waxman to investigate the incidence of physical, sexual, and verbal abuse in nursing homes in the

United States. The investigation found that incidence of abuse violations during annual state inspections has risen dramatically (U.S. House of Representatives, 2001; also see Waxman, 2001). The report cited that the percentage of nursing homes cited for abuse violations has almost tripled since 1996. In 1996, 5.9% of all nursing homes were cited for an abuse violation during their annual inspections. The percentage of homes cited for abuse has risen in each successive year. In 2000, 16.0 % of nursing homes were cited for an abuse violation during their annual inspection.

Nursing Home Abuse in the Bay Area

Due to a recent attempt to address growing concerns regarding elder abuse in nursing homes, the minority staff of the Congressional Government Reform Committee was asked by nine Bay Area members of Congress to investigate the conditions in nursing homes in the San Francisco Bay Area, which comprises the San Francisco, Oakland, San Jose, Vallejo, and Santa Rosa metropolitan areas. There are 288 nursing homes in the Bay Area that accept residents covered by Medicare and Medicaid programs. These homes serve approximately 22,000 residents. This investigation has resulted in a report to evaluate their compliance with federal nursing home standards (House of Government Reform Committee, 2000).

The report finds that there are serious deficiencies in many Bay Area nursing homes and fewer than four percent comply with federal standards. Only 18 out of 288 nursing homes in the Bay Area were in full or substantial compliance with federal standards during their most recent annual inspection. In contrast, 119 nursing homes in the Bay Area – more than one out of three—*had violations that caused actual harm to residents or placed*

11

them at risk of death or serious injury (House of Government Reform Committee, 2000).

Due to the recognition of elder abuse as a national tragedy in the United States, hearings have been conducted before the Subcommittee on Human Services of the House Select Committee on Aging which indicated that 1 out of 25 Americans over the age of 65 suffers from some form of abuse, neglect, or exploitation (U.S. Congress, House Subcommittee on Human Services, 1989). As our elder population increases, we can logically expect that incidents of elder abuse will also increase, if all other variables remain constant.

The problem of rampant abuse in nursing homes is further documented in a recent report on Nursing Home Conditions in the San Francisco Bay Area conducted by the Committee on Government Reform in June 2000, which summarizes some examples of serious quality care problems:

- A male nurse aide molested two elderly female residents by putting his finger in their vaginas while bathing them (State Citation, 1999).

- A nurse aide entered a resident's room and found another staff member on top of the resident with his pants down and the resident's legs spread (State Citation, 1999).

- A 77 -year old resident told inspectors that a nurse aide had pulled her hair, slapped her face, and threw a soiled wet diaper at her head. The aide held the resident's arm so tight that the arm starting bleeding (State Citation, 1999).

- When the resident complained that she was "bleeding to death," the aide said, "Good. I hope you do." (State Citation, 1999).

- A 78- year old resident developed a Stage III pressure sore on her left hip and Stage IV sore on her left foot. As a result of the facility's failure to properly treat the sores, the resident's left leg had to be amputated (State Citation, 1999).

- An 83- year old resident had ants crawling on her face, moving in and out of her mouth, in the bed and food tray (State Citation, 1999).

- A 61 -year old diabetic resident was admitted to a facility following leg surgery. Contrary to the physician orders, the facility failed to provide insulin to the resident for four days and failed to monitor the blood circulation in his leg. As a result, the resident went into a diabetic coma, and his leg had to be amputated (State Citation, 1999).

- Inspectors found that a facility had failed to monitor a resident's feeding tube. As a result, the resident was overfed and later died of cardiopulmonary arrest and aspiration pneumonia (State Citation, 1999).

- The shocking CBS News story of Helen Love who suffered a *broken neck* at the hands of a male certified nurse's assistant angered because she soiled herself. "He choked me and went and broke my neck and broke by wrist", said Love. She died two days after the interview (CBS Health Watch, 2001).

What is Institutional Elder Abuse?

Definitions of institutional elder abuse vary among the states, but the National Aging Resource Center on Elder Abuse has suggested the following working definition for institutional elder abuse: "all forms of maltreatment of older people (60 or 65 years of age and older depending on the state program) that takes place in institutional settings (instead of a domestic or home setting), (Toshio, 1992). Institutional elder abuse refers to the maltreatment of an older person residing in a residential facility for older persons, e.g., a nursing home, board and care home, foster home, or group home (Administration on Aging, 1998). Perpetrators of institutional elder abuse usually are persons who have a legal or contractual obligation to provide care and protection; however, residents can also abuse other residents (DHHS, 1999).

Type of Abuses

Institutional elder abuse can occur in an infinite number of forms. The Office of the Inspector General of the Department of Health and Human Services (OIG) has identified different types of elder abuse found among nursing home residents (Office of the Inspector General, 1990). The OIG has provided the following definitions and examples:

Physical Abuse: The most prevalent form of elder abuse that is reported is physical abuse. Physical abuse is the infliction of any physical pain or injury upon an elder by a person who has care or custody with that elder. It can also be described as any act of violence or rough treatment, whether or not actual physical injury results.

Sexual Abuse: One of the most atrocious offenses perpetrated against the elderly is one of a sexual nature. Abuse is any sexual behavior directed toward an older adult without her or his full knowledge and informed consent. According to a 1991 study conducted by Dr. Holly-Ramsey-Klawsnik, the most prevalent sexual offense involving the elderly is rape (Todd, 1991).

Misuse of Restraints: Chemical or physical control of a resident beyond physician's orders or not in accordance with accepted medical practice. Examples include staff failing to loosen the restraints with adequate time frames or attempting to cope with resident's behavior by inappropriate use of a drug.

Verbal/Emotional Abuse: Infliction of mental/emotional suffering. Examples include demeaning statements, harassment, threats, humiliation or intimidation of the resident.

Physical Neglect: Disregard for necessities of daily living. For example: failure to provide necessary food clothing, clean linens or daily care of the resident's necessities such as brushing a resident's hair, helping with a resident's bath and incontinent care.

Financial Abuse: Any improper conduct, with or without the informed consent of the older adult, that results in a monetary or personal gain to the abuser and/ or personal loss for the older adult.

Medical Neglect: Lack of care for existing medical problems. For example: ignoring a necessary special diet, failure to contact a physician as necessary, lack of awareness of medication side effects, or failure to treat a medical problem.

Medical Abuse: Any medical procedure or treatment that is done without the permission of the older person or their legally recognized proxy. It also refers to actions that are not within accepted medical practice.

Verbal/Emotional Neglect: Creating situations in which esteem is not fostered. For example: failure to consider a resident's wishes, restricting contact with family, friends or other residents, or simply, ignoring the resident's need for verbal and emotional contact.

Personal Property Abuse (Material Goods): Illegal or improper use of a resident's property by another for personal gain. For example: theft of a resident's private television, false teeth, clothing, or jewelry.

Abandonment: The desertion of an individual receiving service at a hospital, nursing facility or similar institution by any person who has assumed responsibility for providing care or by a person who has physical custody of that individual.

Violation of Civil/Human Rights: denial of an older adult's basic rights according to the United Nations Declaration of the Rights of Older Persons.

Signs and Symptoms of Abuse and Neglect

There may be a higher incidence of injury and/or death resulting from physical abuse due to the vulnerability of individual receiving services (Reno, 200). The following signs and symptoms of abuse and neglect are examples of possible indicators of abuse:

- Bruises, black eyes, welts, lacerations, rope marks, imprint injuries
- Fractures*
- Open wounds, cuts, punctures
- Sprains or dislocations
- Unexplained venereal disease or genital infections
- Unexplained vaginal or anal bleeding
- Bruises around the breast or genital area

Factors that Lead to Institutional Elder Abuse

It is important to stress that because something may be described, as a 'cause' of abuse or neglect does not make the abusive act excusable. There is no excuse for an abusive act (Hudson et al, 1991).

16

A primary explanation for abuse from researchers and advocacy groups is that staff are overworked, underpaid and understaffed. In July 1998, Professor Charlene Harrington of the University of California-San Francisco, a leading nursing home expert, found that the current level of nursing home staffing is "completely inadequate to provide care and supervision" (Harrington, 1998). The risk of mistreatment for vulnerable residents in nursing facilities are primarily due to problems of low wages, staff shortages, inadequate training and supervision, poor working conditions, and high staff turnover (Jones, 1997).

According to Lisa Hubbard, spokeswoman for the Service Employees International Union, "Nurses aides are tremendously underpaid and understaffed working in some nursing homes with annual turnover rates that exceed 80 percent. Because of short staffing, nurse's aides often suffer sprains and back trouble from having to shower, lift, turn and sometimes struggle with residents single-handedly (Nurse Week, 2000). Bureau of labor statistics show that back injuries are most frequently reported among nurses' aides. Short tenure and high turnover are correlated with health and safety problems (Personick, 1990).

Some of the violations cited by state inspectors were the result of staff shortages. At one facility, the staff stopped coming to work because their paychecks were bouncing. When inspectors visited the home, they found only four staff members caring for 69 residents. Inspectors described the scene as chaotic and unorganized. Numerous residents were left in feces and urine-soaked clothes all day, and one resident was found wandering outside the facility. Inspectors also found that the home's administrator did not have a clear idea of how many staff would be reporting on a daily basis (State Citation, 1999).

Routines in institutions are seen as important, and residents who do not cooperate may cause frustration in workers, who react in anger (Bourget, 1999). Faced with heavier levels of care, difficulties in caring for impaired and dependent residents and stress from dealing with residents with debilitating diseases cause aggravation, which is often taken out on residents (Frolik, 1995). Employees and labor organizations argue that low wages, especially for nurses' aides and orderlies cause high turnover and low morale, which leads to elder abuse (Service Employee, 1990).

A provision of nursing home law known as the "Boren Amendment "guarantees that nursing homes would receive "reasonable and adequate" Medicaid reimbursements to provide quality care. Since the repeal of the Boren Amendment, there is evidence suggesting that Medicaid reimbursement rates have not kept pace with the rising costs of providing nursing home care (Department of Health and Human Services, 2000). Nursing homes have argued that lower Medicaid reimbursement rates have made it more difficult for them to recruit and retain quality staff (American Health Care Association, 2000)

Four Factors Studies

Complimenting the work described above, Pillemer and Bennett (1993) have identified four specific factors that may lead to institutional elder abuse: exogenous (external factors), nursing home environment, staff characteristics, and patient characteristics.

1. Exogenous Factors- there are two factors external to the care of the facility in particular that may lead to abuse: supply and demand of facility beds and the unemployment rate. First, if the area has a surplus of beds, patients may be accepted without adequate assessment, resulting in misplacement. Where there is a shortage of beds, patients may be forced into facilities with reputations for poor care. Secondly, the unemployment rate along with rates of pay affects the staffing

levels of facilities.

2. Nursing Home Environment- Homes oriented towards custodial care often experience more abusive situations. Other environmental factors include the physical design of the building, the level of care sustained by the facility, size, rates, and costs of care, the staff-patient ratio, and turnover rate of both patients and staff.

3. Staff Characteristics- Typically, staff members who abuse patients can be described as young males that lack experience. They are often poorly educated and suffer from job burnout, which is defined as physical, emotional and spiritual exhaustion and ultimately involves loss of concern for the patients.

4. Patient Characteristics- Many patients who find themselves victims of abuse are mentally[1] or physically incapacitated, thus leading to more stress on the caregiver. Additionally, victims lack regular visitors who can watch for abusive situations.

---

[1] Indeed, the rates of psychiatric disorders in nursing homes have been estimated to be at least 50% to 94% of the population; these residents are in need of mental health consultation, which is often withheld. It is likely that widespread overuse and misuse of psychoactive medications add to the psychological woes of nursing home residents (Senior-Site, 1990).

Abuse of Residents Is a Major Problem in U.S Nursing Homes

The state inspection reports and citations documented that many residents were subjected to serious physical abuse by nursing home staff. This physical abuse caused numerous injuries, including a fractured femur, a fractured hip, a fractured elbow, severe bruises, lacerations of the head, neck and hands, bruises to the eye and bruises to the thigh, a fractured wrist, a fractured thumb, and a variety of other injuries (HFCA, 1999). The state inspection report included all forms of abuse documented in previous chapters and concluded that abuse of nursing home residents is a widespread and significant problem involving serious abuses that cause significant damage to the health and well-being of nursing home residents (HFCA, 2000).

Current Laws, Legislation and Strategies

All states have passed laws governing elder abuse reporting. In 42 states including California such reporting is mandatory for human service professionals (healthcare practitioners, social workers, clergy, teachers, government agents and law enforcement officials) who come in contact with the elderly. Reporting is done voluntarily in Colorado, Illinois, Wisconsin, New York, Pennsylvania, North and South Dakota, and New Jersey (Capezuti, 1997). Most states require individuals to report evidence that leads them to "reasonably believe" that the elderly person in question is the victim of abuse or neglect.

To protect the confidentiality and beneficent intent of the reporter, in addition to eliminating concerns of retribution and liability, all states provide good faith immunity for the reporter, regardless of whether abuse is confirmed. In many states, healthcare professionals who report abuse are also protected by "disclosure confidentiality" laws, which forbid the disclosure of the identity of the reporter without that individual's written consent (National Center on Elder Abuse, 1997).

All fifty states and the District of Columbia have enacted legislation authorizing the provision of adult protective services (APS) in cases of elder abuse. Generally, these APS laws establish a system for the reporting and investigation of elder abuse and for the provision of social services to help the victim and ameliorate the abuse. In most jurisdictions, these laws pertain to abused adults who have a disability/vulnerability/impairment as defined by state law, not just to older persons (Adult Protective Services, 2001). There are APS state laws that identify individuals who reside in long-term care facilities (known as "institutional abuse"). Like the APS laws, institutional abuse statutes create a mechanism for reporting, investigating and addressing incidents of elder abuse that occur in long-term care facilities (LTCF's) or other facilities covered under the law (American Bar Association, 1998).

Adult Protective Services provides service through the state social service department. They receive and screen calls for potential seriousness and typically operate a hotline available 24 hours a day, 7 day a week for a concerned citizen or a practicing professional serving the elderly who suspect that abuse has occurred or is occurring to an older person. If a suspected incident involves an older person living in an institutional setting, anyone concerned about the resident's safety is encouraged to call the office of the local long-term care (LTC) ombudsman (Administration on Aging, 1998). Reports of abuse that occur in a nursing home, a board and care home, a residential facility for the elderly, or at a long-term care facility are the responsibility of the Ombudsman's office, which is administered by The California Department of Aging.

In 1965, the Older Americans Act was enacted to protect vulnerable adults and provides state Area Agencies on Aging to assess the need for elder abuse prevention services. The Administration on Aging within the Department of Health and Human Services, under the Old Americans Act, established the Long-Term Care Ombudsman program that began 25years ago (Cherry, 1993). They have thousands of paid and volunteer ombudsmen working in every state who advocate on behalf of individuals and groups of residents as well as to effect system changes on local, state and national levels. They provide an ongoing presence in long-term care facilities, monitoring care and conditions and providing a voice for those who are unable to speak for themselves (Cherry, 1993). Long-term ombudsmen report directly to Adult Protective Services.

Any nursing home that receives federal funding must comply with federal nursing home laws that Congress enacted in 1987, known as the Nursing Home Reform Act, which requires that nursing homes " provide services and activities to attain or maintain the highest practicable physical, mental and psychological well-being of each resident in accordance to a written care plan" (Smith, 2001).

Legislation has not led to clear and consistent implementation of policy by health facility inspectors. Inspectors that evaluate nursing homes have varying opinions and interpretations of the elder abuse reporting procedures, which can cause discrepancies in identifying abuse. In order to better understand the process for reporting, an investigation of the state public health department procedures for reporting elder abuse was initiated via an exploratory study conducted between April and October 1989 (Ehrlich, 1989). A brief two-page questionnaire was mailed to State health department directors. A cover letter identified the purposes of the study, requested their cooperation with an immediate response, and promised to provide them with a report on the findings.

The letter also identified the staff members of the health departments as "front –line workers who can make a significant contribution to the early identification of abuse situations". All 50 States responded. The respondents who completed the questionnaires had varying disciplines and staff responsibilities within the health departments or were from agencies that the State had designated to investigate elder abuse. Two follow-up mailings to non-respondents plus five telephone interviews resulted in a response rate of 100 percent (Ehrlich, 1989).

The questionnaire, entitled "Survey of State Health Departments on Elder Abuse Reporting Procedures," collected data in the following areas:

- Administrative awareness of the State law for reporting elder abuse and neglect,

- Procedures developed by the State health departments to assure compliance with the law by health care practitioners,

- Awareness and identification of difficulties encountered by health personnel in reporting situations of abuse and neglect.

The results of the study revealed five common mistakes made by people trained by the State Health Departments to follow procedures on elder abuse reporting. The results are:

1. Awareness of the law: 47 responded yes. 3 states responded no. Of the three States responding "No" to the awareness of the law, all three have laws with mandatory professional reporting requirements.

2. Procedures-- department written protocols. There were 38 respondents who reported that their health department had *no protocol* specifically prepared for staff members or related community professionals.

3. More than half (18) of them indicated that it was not the responsibility of their department. Comments of the six other State respondents suggest a range of

   attitudes on the subject. Ten health departments responded that they had department protocols.

4. Procedures—department training programs. There were 14 respondents who indicated that their departments conducted training or awareness campaigns, or both, for physicians and nurses at the time the law was implemented. Six departments maintain ongoing in-service, particularly to clarify legal requirements.

5. Reporting difficulties. Less than one-third of the respondents said they knew of difficulties encountered by health care practitioners in reporting abuse. This group of respondents identified a number of general reporting issues applicable to the total reporting system as well as to the health professional.

Further findings indicate that the State Health Department employees trained to report elder abuse lacked clarity of the law—limited familiarity with the requirements, procedures, investigative agencies, and differences between reporting community-based and long-term care facility abuse. The questionnaire results revealed the following areas of discrepancies:

- Different definitions of abuse used by health department staff members and abuse investigators,
- Lack of adequate number of investigators and timely investigations,

- Lack of public awareness,
- Uneasiness about reporting—professional denial of abuse occurrence or the unwillingness of families to cooperate, or both, and
- Lack of confidentiality for the person reporting abuse.

The findings suggest that State departments of health are aware of elder abuse reporting laws, but it appears that little has been done to further their implementation. More specifically, none of the 50 departments of health surveyed has developed an actual protocol around abuse identification and referral. Sixty-four percent also lacked related in-service training of health care providers, and nearly three- fourths offered no awareness campaign regarding the law (Ehrlich, 1989). To better understand the policy context in terms of funding, federal law states that nursing homes that receive Medicaid and Medicare funds must meet federal standards of care. This law requires that nursing homes "provide services and activities to attain or maintain the highest practicable physical, mental, and psychological well-being of each resident." The overwhelming majority of nursing homes in the United States receive funding through either the Medicaid program or the Medicare program, or both (HFCA, 1998).

My background and the Black church: An appropriate setting for the C.A.P.
Locating the C.A.P. program within Allen Temple church is in keeping with the churches role as an engine for social change. The U.S. Census reports that there are 36 million African-Americans, approximately nine million African-American families and four million African-Americans with degrees. There are 85,000 African American churches that receive three billion annually and possess $50 billion in assets (Jawanza, 2003). These statistics are notable to the strength and role of the churches ability to affect social change in the African-American community. Indeed, during my early childhood I was taken to Allen Temple Baptist Church to participate in what my parents called " a spiritual growth experience" that prepared me to be concerned about the well being of others, especially seniors. In our home and in the church, I was taught that seniors are special and should be treated with dignity and respect. I was raised to be considerate of seniors, respect the church and listen attentively to the pastor.

Our pastor, Dr. J. Alfred Smith Sr. would preach sermons about the historical role of the Black church in caring for seniors and shared countless stories about his grandmother,

Amy, who helped raise him. The Black pastor has almost limitless opportunities to cause critically needed social change (Forrest, 1993). He emphasized the responsibility of Allen Temple in meeting the needs of seniors who are unable to attend church, seniors that live in long-term care settings and seniors that are sick who need the churches support. Allen Temple owns and operates five senior retirement communities and groups of church members are assigned to visit them when they become sick and shut-in, taking them communion and providing companionship to those seniors. Moral accountability is inseparably linked to the ethics and values inherent in the aspirations and hopes of the black church and community (Forrest, 1993). The pastor organized activities that focuses on senior care in the church and the community and accentuated how we should treasure, honor and respect them as "senior saints".

Similar to church teachings, my parents also taught my siblings and me that it was our responsibility to care for those less fortunate than we and for the protection and caring of seniors. Protest against injustice is a familiar action of the Black community through the church (Smith, 1982). Living by example, my father moved his elderly mother from Texarcana, Arkansas into our home in California so that we could take care of her. She lived with us until she became very ill and required a higher level of care in a nursing home. My family took turns sitting at her bedside so that she would never wake up or be alone in this nursing home setting. In retrospect, I realized that the Care Advocate Program (C.A.P.) is an extension of my spirit and determination to protect seniors from elder abuse in an institutional setting that had been unknowingly established in my formative years.

My siblings and I were the only Black girls in the elementary school we attended and only a few Black families lived in our neighborhood. My mother, Dr. Carolyn Stuckey, would sit us down and discuss the Civil and Human Rights Movement. She would read stories to us about the Civil Rights Movement and required us to watch footage televised on history channels that taught us about Martin Luther King, Jr. She was adamant about teaching us where we as a people came from, what we as a people had to suffer and how we could and should excel past the difficult circumstances Black people shared. Both my parents were raised in the South and my mother was born to bi-racial parents during a time when Blacks and Whites were discouraged from being married. The racial discrimination and oppression that they experienced living in the South may have been the springboard for their parenting teaching and practices. According to our parents, we were to know and believe that we could reach the highest pillar of personal, social and academic excellence and that we should embrace civil and human rights for everyone.

The C.A.P. program is organized through the church and rooted in the belief that all people have the human right to be treated with dignity and respect. Liberation implies a quality of life that honors the inherent dignity and worth of all persons (Smith, 1982). The Care Advocate Program is a model for caring for seniors that promotes a friendly visiting service from trained and knowledgeable volunteers working with the church to ensure quality care and protection of seniors in long-term care settings where abuse is rampant. It was Martin Luther King Jr., who made the contemporary church aware of its power to affect change. King developed a theory and practice that Blacks had both a moral right and responsibility to disobey unjust laws in their resistance to social evils (Walter, 1976). Allen Temple Baptist church has established collaboration with the

C.A.P. program in an effort to provide protection to seniors living in a nursing home who may be subjected to abuse or neglect. I consider the abuse of a senior by caregivers as a social evil and sought the strength of the church to provide a means by which a designated team of trained volunteers could monitor the care received, report abuse if found and advocate for the senior and their families in these settings.

The Care Advocate Program is based in the church and seeks to respond to the social and health care crisis that seniors face commonly known as "The Hidden Terror". The goal of community, as expressed in the Black Christian tradition, is to create a world of "non-oppression" that supports the liberation of all persons for participation in God's freedom, justice and love. The hallmark of Martin Luther King Jr., prophetic ministry, "The theology of Civil Rights Era" underscored the role of the Black church as a historically conscious liberation community. During the King era, Black churches and social hope of the Black community were united (Forrest, 1997).

Allen Temple and the Care Advocate Program are addressing the terror that seniors are quietly suffering by developing a group of knowledgeable participants that are courageous and trained to confront elder abuse with support from protective service agencies and informed involved families.

III. CARE ADVOCATE PROGRAM CONCEPTUAL FRAMEWORK

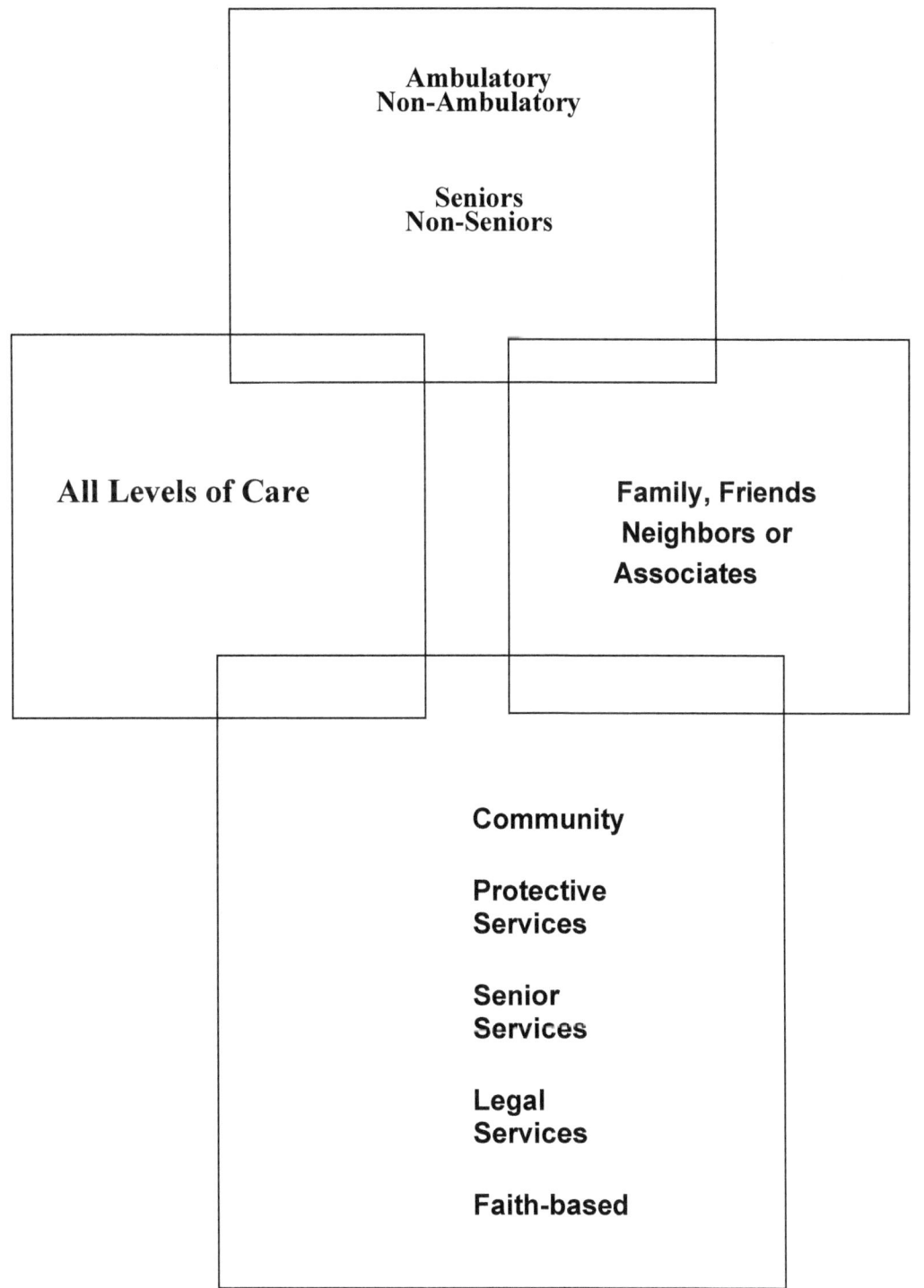

Ambulatory
Non-Ambulatory

Seniors
Non-Seniors

All Levels of Care

Family, Friends
Neighbors or
Associates

Community

Protective
Services

Senior
Services

Legal
Services

Faith-based

Figure I: Care Advocate Program Curriculum Overview

CARE ADVOCATE PROGRAM

Training Day I:

Complete a pre-test

Watch videotape on nursing home abuse

Understand the characteristics of domestic and institutional elder abuse

Learn how to intervene and report abuse

Understand the legal and legislative process

Interact with representatives from elder abuse protection agencies

Training Day II:

Learn about medical conditions that affect seniors

Understand the characteristics of physical and sexual abuse from physicians Learn about physical limitations, functional impairments and use of assistive devices

Review the affects of immobility and the causes of skin breakdown

Understand nutritional health and deficiencies

Interact with medical doctors and a nutritionist

Training Day III:

Review the C.A.P. training manual

Understand the state survey process

Learn how to access the Internet for information about nursing homes

Understand how to advocate on behalf of seniors and their families

Participate in role-playing and nursing home simulation exercises

Prepare for facility site visits

IV. METHODS

Intervention: Description of the Care Advocate Program

The Care Advocate Program (C.A.P.) is a comprehensive training series designed to address elder abuse in institutional settings by:

- Educating participants about the characteristics of institutional elder abuse.
- Providing effective techniques for interfacing with protective service agencies.
- Training participants to use proactive intervention strategies.
- Teaching participants methods for advocating on behalf of nursing home residents and their families.

The Care Advocate Program's goal is to provide trainees with a clear understanding of elder abuse reporting, prevention and protection systems. The Care Advocate Program required trainees to attend three consecutive Saturdays of four- hour classroom training and perform four facility site visits to an Allen Temple member residing in a nursing home. Trainees completed a sequence of questionnaires intended to help address the effectiveness of C.A.P. and evaluate areas of program improvement. (See Figure 1 for summary of program design).

Training Day I

The first day of C.A.P. training was held in a large conference room in the Family Life Center at Allen Temple Baptist Church. The goal of the first training session was to educate trainees about institutional elder abuse and introduce them to representatives from elder abuse reporting agencies and protective groups with whom they would work. It *was* crucial to the success of the Care Advocate Program that trainees establish a rapport and collaborate with the state organizations responsible for responding when abuse *was* reported.

Observing elder abuse or neglect in a nursing home setting can be a frightening experience and trainees needed to be empowered to act on suspected abuse by advocating on behalf of the resident. The session began with a pre-test for participants. (See Figure A.) The pre-test was collected, participants were greeted and paneled guest were seated with lapel microphones. Once everyone was settled, I introduced each paneled guest, gave a brief description of the organizations they represent and explained their role in working with the Care Advocate Program. There were seven guests that represented the following agencies; Adult Protective Services, Ombudsman, California Advocates for Nursing Home Reform, Alameda County District Attorney's Office and the City of Oakland's Police Departments Elder Abuse Division.

The problem of elder abuse in nursing homes is often difficult to imagine and many find it hard to believe that the abuse of a frail senior by paid caregivers is real. In order to bring reality to this problem, I show videotape from a Channel 2 television special news report on Nursing Home Abuse in the Bay Area featuring reporters Dennis Richmond and Leslie Griffith. This news report interviews experts and advocates on nursing home abuse with personal testimonies from seniors who have suffered abuse in a nursing home setting. One of the seniors featured in this news report had her wrist and neck broken by the nurse caring for her. She died two days after the interview. Once the videotape was completed, participants sat in silence with tears in their eyes shaking their head in disbelief. A brief question and answer period was provided to allow participants an opportunity to discuss what was viewed on the news report.

The Care Advocate Program strives to provide a holistic approach to addressing institutional abuse by introducing representatives from five organizations that work in different ways, to protect seniors residing in these settings. The C.A.P. trainees received a thirty-minute presentation from each panelist who shared descriptive information about the characteristics of elder abuse, proper procedures for notifying their particular office and techniques for ensuring resident safety without placing them at risk for further abuse. Trainees were given brochures, flyers and handouts with toll-free contact numbers of the protective agencies they could contact if abuse or neglect was suspected. This was followed by a presentation from Adult Protective Services (A.P.S.). This is the organization responsible for investigating abuse, neglect and exploitation of adults who are elderly or have disabilities living at home.

It is crucial that C.A.P. trainees understand the role of APS and receives information about domestic abuse seniors often suffer at the hands of family, friends and neighbors. Trainees were educated about the "cycle of abuse" that occurs when seniors are victims of domestic abuse and are then subjected to abuse in the nursing home. This can potentially lead to a senior remaining silent and afraid to tell of the abuse because a nursing home staff member is now perpetrating it. The APS representative provided a detailed power point presentation on elder abuse and neglect and gave each participant a laminated elder abuse and prevention fact sheet that trainees could use for future reference.

The next step was to introduce C.A.P. trainees to the Ombudsman Program. Trainees will interface with this program more than any other because they are the agency designated to investigate elder abuse complaints in nursing homes. It is a mandated state law that information regarding Ombudsman should be posted, wheelchair level, in the lobby of every licensed nursing home. When trainees conduct their site visits, they looked for the Ombudsman sign as part of their facility evaluation. The glaring problem with this mandate is that if a senior is sick, isolated and abused, they are unable to see a sign in the lobby or have the ability to follow through. The C.A.P. trainee is to contact the Ombudsman if abuse is suspected and follow-up on the abuse reporting process on behalf of the senior. The representative from the Ombudsman program provided educational materials on elder abuse and neglect found specifically in a nursing home environment with contact numbers to access protective services.

I felt it imperative to emphasize the Ombudsman program and their role in responding to C.A.P. trainees because this agency is responsible for investigating and resolving complaints made by, or on behalf of, individual residents in these settings. Trainees could potentially witness nursing home abuse during their facility site visits and must understand the "fear of retaliation" that seniors may experience. This fear can cause seniors and their families to be very afraid to tell that abuse is occurring because the abuser will abuse more if exposed. All too often, Ombudsman and any other protective service agency may never know a nursing home resident is being abused due to the fear of retaliation or code of silence. This is the primary reason why it is so important to have C.A.P. trainees visit the nursing home facility, establish a rapport with the potentially abused senior and advocate on their behalf when they are too scared or at risk to do it alone.

Ombudsmen receive constant complaints about inadequate nurse- patient staffing ratios in nursing homes. The shortage causes staff frustration and leads to abuse because they are not able to do their jobs properly. One of the key methods of initiating significant change in nursing home staffing patterns is for C.A.P. trainees to become part of the legal and legislative process of improving care. Thus, a representative from California Advocates for Nursing Home Reform (C.A.N.H.R.) educated trainees about the legislative process that enacts public policy. California Advocates for Nursing Home Reform is a non-profit information and advocacy organization dedicated to improving the quality of care and quality of life for nursing home residents, their families and their friends through community education, legislation and litigation. It is important that C.A.P. trainees understand the legal and legislative process that was presented by C.A.H.N.R. because this is the primary means by which to demand accountability and assurances of better care in a nursing home setting.

The Care Advocate Program emphasizes the need for accountability and resident safety. Trainees, therefore, received moving presentations from representatives with the Alameda County District Attorney's Elder Abuse Division office who communicated a clear message that the abusive conduct from perpetrators is serious, illegal and will not be tolerated. The District Attorney's Office plays a significant role in fighting abuse and improving the quality of life for seniors and has established an easy access senior program. Representatives of this office educated the trainees about elder abuse laws, methods of reporting to the access program and systems established to defend seniors in a court of law. If abuse is suspected and charges are filed against the perpetrator, it is the DA's office that will pursue litigation and trainees may be asked to testify on behalf of the abused senior. So it was good to familiarize them with this office as well.

At this time, trainees viewed disturbing power point presentations with graphic photos of seniors who had been physically and sexually abused, neglected and assaulted in nursing homes. Trainees viewed pictures of seniors that were left lying in their own waste and severely neglected with bruises, open wounds and fractures caused by facility staff. Trainee became tearful while observing these photographed images of the physical abuse and neglect nursing home residents suffer. Both district attorneys emphasized that silence and fear of reporting abusive staff members has become a common reality in nursing homes and the presence of C.A.P. trainees can make a difference. The Care Advocate Program prepares trainees to understand abuse of seniors by providing information that includes:

- Types of elder abuse
- Causes of abuse
- Victim profiles
- Abuser profiles
- Physical indicators
- Behavioral indicators of the victim

- Indicators from the family/caregiver
- Indications of possible financial abuse

The C.A.P trainees were also presented with cases and scenarios demonstrating how seniors were being taken for granted and having their money stolen as a result of fraud, deception and criminal tactics by perpetrators. They received information on how to protect seniors from fraudulent activities, methods of securing their finances and steps taken to report financial abuse if suspected. Trainees learned about the characteristics of the perpetrator who masters the game of swindling, defrauding and coning people out of their financial resources. Given that perpetrators can be described as a friendly and charming person that befriends the trusting senior and someone who they would least suspect, the trainees were educated to recognize the perpetrator in a nursing home setting. They are typically the paid caregivers employed by the facility.

Trainees learned about situational scenarios of financial abuse experienced by seniors in a nursing home that include:

- Changes in bank practice
- Unauthorized ATM withdrawals
- Addition of names to a bank signature card
- Sudden changes in a will
- Disappearance of funds or possessions
- Unpaid bills despite financial resources

The C.A.P. trainees were presented with the following vignettes for discussion:

Vignette #1: A 90- year- old man who had been left lying in his own waste, not fed for days, covered with infected unattended bedsores and severely neglected in a nursing home located in Oakland.

Vignette#2: An 85-year-old woman who had been sodomized and choked by the nursing assistant care for her in a local nursing home. He left fingerprint bruises around her neck and caused broken blood vessels in the back of her throat from the impact of sexual abuse.

Vignette #3: A 90-year- old widowed male left credit cards, identification and money in a safe secured in the administrative offices of the nursing home facility. A nurse with access to the locked area stole them and made withdrawals from the account.

The C.A.P. trainees engaged in a brief question and answer period about the vignettes to become familiar with examples of abuse that they may face when conducting facility site visits. The first training day concluded with a presentation from the Oakland Police Department's Elder Abuse Division. This division provides the community with police officers that have received special training to respond and investigate complaints of elder abuse. Trainees were shown front-page newspaper articles that describe nursing home abuse as the "Hidden Terror". The police officer explained that when it was time for trainees to visit the nursing homes, they should always remember that the visit is just like an iceberg. The part of an iceberg that is visible can be likened to the every day routine of a nursing home setting but the part of the iceberg that is hidden can conceal abuse that goes undetected and underreported. The C.A.P. trainees were educated about the collaboration efforts that occur between Police officers, District Attorney's, Ombudsman and Adult Protective Services with emphasis on their role in working closely with the Care Advocate Program to expose this Hidden Terror.

The first day of training ended with a reception to allow trainees an opportunity to ask additional questions and interact with paneled guest. The C.A.P. trainees were given educational materials, fliers, pamphlets, pens, pads, brochures and business cards from each guest that they could use as resource guides.

Training Day II

The second day of C.A.P. training was held in the Studio Room in the Family Life Center. The goal of the second training session was to educate trainees about the physical, sexual, emotional and nutritional effects of elder abuse that seniors could suffer in an institutional setting. It began with presentations by a panel of clinicians who are well known in the Oakland community, have a long history of professional practices and have received awards and honors for excellent service. This session provided an opportunity for C.A.P. trainees to enhance their knowledge about the signs and symptoms of abuse that they could potentially observe from a team of medical doctors and a licensed dietician. Trainees learned in classroom sessions that urinary tract infections, infected bedsores, dehydration and malnutrition are the leading cause of resident deaths in a nursing home. It is vital to the success of this program to provide trainees, who may not be familiar with medical issues, information about specific indicators of abuse that they can apply when visiting and observing their assigned facility.

An Internist and recognized television talk show host who has a private medical practice provided trainees with clinical information about age-specific diagnoses that cause seniors to be admitted to a nursing home. Trainees were educated about common medical conditions of seniors including; coronary artery disease (heart problems), diabetes (endocrine problems), chronic constipation (intestinal problems), degenerative joint disease (arthritic problems), cerebral vascular accidents (neurological problems), peripheral vascular disease (circulation problems) and cataracts/glaucoma (visual problems) to name a few. Trainees will repeatedly see these medical conditions because they consistently affect the senior population. The speaker provided trainees with educational materials about these conditions and taught them about the increased incidence of depression among seniors residing in long-term care facilities.

Depression among the senior population is prevalent in this society. It is a condition that physicians regularly treat seniors prior to and during nursing home admissions. Seniors are lonely, isolated and become depressed when they struggle to navigate through our current complex health care system. The internist explained how seniors find it difficult to obtain necessary medical services when attempting to utilize automated telephone systems, waiting on hold for long periods of time, and unfamiliarity with medical terminology. The C.A.P. trainees were educated about mental health issues and the increased incidence of depression, dementia, and Alzheimer's found in seniors. Trainees will observe seniors with mental health problems when visiting their facilities because these problems are obvious in a nursing home setting.

The second speaker was a prominent Obstetrician/Gynecologist, who is a professor at Stanford University and a medical provider who maintains two private practices in the Oakland community. He focused the discussion on the signs and symptoms of sexual abuse, gynecological conditions and hormonal changes commonly seen with seniors. The C.A.P. trainees were taught about the chief complaints of women who experience symptoms of discomfort related to having night sweats, hot flashes, erratic menstrual cycles and fatigue. Men also experience hormonal imbalances, increased incidence of impotence, urinary and prostrate problems that often go untreated because men are typically hesitant to seek medical care. Hormonal changes can affect both male and female seniors' mental status and cause them to experience short and long-term memory deficits, feelings of depression and dementia.

Care Advocate Program trainees have been taught that sexual abuse of seniors is prevalent in nursing homes and that seniors are frequently faced with the risk of being sexually abused. Trainees were educated about the prevalence of vulnerable seniors being raped, sodomized and sexually assaulted by paid caregivers working in the facility. The Obstetrician/Gynecologist presented trainees with examples of certain types of bruises, skin tears and broken blood vessels that could be the signs and symptoms caused by sexual abuse. It was very hard for the trainees to learn about sexual abuse, no one wants to believe that a nursing home worker would choke, slap, sodomize and rape a senior. Trainees sat stunned and tearful at the end of this presentation. The presenter showed them a picture of his beautiful new baby girl that generated a rhythmic sigh of delight and a short break was taken to decrease group tension and encourage group support.

The next guest was a medical doctor, who recently graduated from Stanford, directs a physical therapy facility and has distinct training as a physiatrist. A physiatrist is a doctor who specializes in movement. He educated C.A.P. trainees about commonly seen functional impairments, physical limitations and use of assistive devices commonly affecting seniors who live in long-term care settings. Seniors are dependent on assistive devices including: wheelchairs, walkers, canes, grab bars, and lifts due to lack of mobility, poor balance and unsteady gait. It was crucial that trainees learn about the mobility changes that occur with seniors and the use of assistive devices that they will inevitably observe during site visits.

Trainees were informed that nursing home staff is mandated by state regulations to turn bed bound seniors every two hours even though they are often left in the same position for extended periods of time lying in their own waste. Because of this, seniors often experience skin breakdown, decubitus ulcers and infections that lead to death related to immobility. Trainees will have the opportunity to observe seniors that are left lying in the bed with no one attempting to help get them up or participate in physical activities. The C.A.P. trainees learned that one of the most common reasons why seniors are treated in an emergency room is due to falls and the most common surgery performed on seniors is hip replacements related to falls. The Physiatrist reviewed common age-related conditions and proactive measures that can be taken to avoid physical decline related to immobility, inactivity and injuries.

Our final guest was a nutritionist for Alameda County Nutrition Services who teaches classes in the community on nutritional health and healthy living. She trains community members and health care providers at community senior centers, senior retirement homes, physicians' offices and television talk shows about nutritional risks and medical conditions related to dietary insufficiencies. The Care Advocate Program focuses a great deal of training on nutrition because seniors are dying from malnutrition and dehydration in nursing care facilities. It is crucial that trainees have knowledge about the characteristics of seniors who are malnourished and dehydrated because this is evidence of abuse and neglect that often leads to resident illness or death.

The C.A.P. trainees reviewed chronic nutritional deficiencies and the dietary recommendations that many seniors are prescribed i.e. low salt, low sugar, low cholesterol or high fiber diet. The nutritionist reviewed the value of taking vitamins and minerals, regular exercise, proper diets and nutritional supplements like Ensure, Glucerna, Boost and Magnacal. The nutritionist used an overhead projector to show pictures of a nutritionally deprived frail seniors sitting in the same chair and being left lying in bed by the nursing home staff. The C.A.P. trainees were taught to visit nursing home residents during mealtimes to become advocates for appropriate and adequate food intake on behalf of vulnerable seniors who often have their food left in front of them with no assistance or deprived of a meal because the nursing staff ate it.

Training Day III

The third day of C.A.P. training was held in the Family Life Center's Health Education Library. The first goal of the third session was to review the Care Advocate Programs'

43

training manual that trainees will use as a reference guide for accessing pertinent elder abuse information. Trainees were seated around an oval conference table with their training manual and participated in a progressive discussion about elder abuse, prevention strategies and reporting guidelines. This process served as a refresher course for trainees to review information presented by the paneled guests in the first two classroom sessions. Trainees reviewed methods of advocating on behalf of the resident and their families and received copies of the Family Communication form that they will use to give feedback to the family once facility site visits are completed.

Trainees requested the opportunity to use time in this third session to give personal testimonies about the impact the program has had on them. The request was of course granted and trainees went around the table candidly expressing their feelings, fears and concerns related to learning that seniors were abused and neglected in nursing homes. This process promoted peer support and cohesiveness. Trainees engaged in dialogue about the inspiration the Care Advocate Program has had on them personally and their commitment to completing all three training sessions with follow-up visits to the nursing home. It was apparent that the elder abuse information had a tremendous affect on them individually and collectively. Tears were shed and feelings expressed about the devastation seniors face and the impact trainees will have on the lives of those visited. A sense of commitment to the families, community and church was a common theme among the trainees.

The second goal of the third training session was to educate trainees about the survey process conducted annually on all licensed nursing homes by the State of California

Department of Health Services' Licensing Division (D.H.S.). Please note: A Department of Health Service's representative was invited to be a C.A.P. presenter but was unable to attend. It is of utmost importance that trainees understand the tremendous impact the Department of Health has on the nursing home industry. Nursing homes are issued facility licenses by the Department of Health and have annual surveys that determine the quality or lack of care received. Allen Temple has a computer lab equipped with high-speed an Internet capability that is located on the second floor of the Family Life Center. Trainees were escorted to the computer lab to learn how to access the Internet for information regarding nursing homes, licensing survey results, elder abuse prevention and educational resources from the D.H.S. web site. Trainees were taught about the procedure used to conduct annual nursing home surveys, the role of health facility evaluators, reviewing licensing survey reports that document quality care deficiencies found during this compliance process.

C.A.P. trainees were educated about state laws that mandate nursing homes to post their annual surveys in the lobby of a facility for anyone to be able to request and review. It is crucial for trainees to be aware of the DHS survey because it gives them a baseline of information about the facility from the trained eye of a licensing evaluator. Health Facility Evaluators are very intelligent, highly trained and profoundly skilled individuals who are typically registered nurses. They have a keen eye for assessing all aspects of quality care rendered to seniors and determining if the facility operation is functioning in compliance to state laws.

The Care Advocate Program emphasizes that one of the main entities that nursing homes immediately respond to is the Department of Health Services. Trainees reviewed what happens when a facility is subjected to this survey process and the operational change often seen when these pre-scheduled surveys occur. Anyone who works in this environment will tell you of the tremendous temporary transformation a nursing home undergoes when the licensing survey process is about to takes place. Trainees were provided with examples of how residents who would normally be left lying in their own waste are all of a sudden dressed, groomed and sitting in the activity room. I shared an experience with trainees of witnessing one nursing home that kept a "survey is coming closet". The closet held paintings, rugs, plants and supplies not ordinarily displayed until the surveyors arrived at the facility.

Trainees expressed concern about visiting the nursing home alone and agreed among them that they would prefer to visit in pairs. They felt that this would provide them with greater support and feedback from a co-trainee to avoid misinterpretation of an unfamiliar environment where abuse may be present. Because there were six volunteers in the C.A.P. training, it was decided that they would be paired and assigned to three different nursing home facilities equipped with educational materials, resource guides and telephone numbers that can be accessed if abuse was suspected. Trainees participated in a simulated nursing home visit through role-playing to prepare them for the visit and increase familiarity with the site visiting process. This marked the end of the three-part classroom training sessions and the beginning of the nursing home site visits to Allen Temple members who gave consent of participation in the Care Advocate Program training.

An Appropriate Setting for this Work: Allen Temple

The Care Advocate Program training was conducted at Allen Temple Baptist Church (A.T.B.C.) in the Family Life Center. I chose to conduct the research study at Allen Temple because I have been a member there since the age of 9 and the pastor of the church, Dr. J. Alfred Smith Sr., has been my godfather since I was 12 years old. My siblings and I were raised in this church and many who are now seniors were instrumental in my growth and development during formative years. I had a conference with my godfather and discussed institutional elder abuse and how seniors are being physically, sexually, financially and emotionally abused and neglected in long-term care settings.

With Dr. Smith's encouragement, I decided that my doctoral research study would be completed at Allen Temple because it would be greatly supported by the congregation many of whom have known me since childhood. Allen Temple has been a pioneer in making community-wide efforts to reach out to seniors for spiritual, social, housing and health-related support and resources. The Care Advocate Program and the Allen Temple church are collaborating to respond to the needs of seniors who are at risk for abuse living in nursing homes. Allen Temple provided the C.A.P. program with the resources needed for media equipment, catered food, conference spaces and the use of a computer lab.

Under the dynamic leadership of the pastor, Dr. J. Alfred Smith Sr., Allen Temple Baptist Church owns and operates numerous senior retirement communities and has a large populace of seniors in the church membership. Allen Temple has played a key role in providing over 25 community and family-oriented programs and services. Dr. J. Alfred Smith Sr. is the author of 16 books has earned over 125 awards and was named the Outstanding Citizen of the Year by the Oakland Tribune. Dr. Keith Russell, President of The American Baptist Seminary of the West, recently announced that the fourth floor assembly room at the seminary would be named in his honor.

Allen Temple has initiated partnerships with organizations that offer health and social services to the community. Pacific Gas and Electric collaborated with Allen Temple to create an Energy Partners Senior Care Program assisting older adults with financial support for high-cost utility bills and a varied host of free utility services. Allen Temple collaborates with the Alzheimer's Association to provide a God's Safe Return Program for seniors who become lost and cannot find there way home due to the ill effects of Alzheimer's. Allen Temple has also been awarded a grant from the Susan B. Kromer Foundation for a Breast Cancer Early Detection and Treatment Program that will be located on the church campus that will provide service to three counties.

Allen Temple has recently built a 25 unit housing facility for persons suffering with AIDS or has been diagnosed as HIV positive. The opening of this facility was personally visited and supported by Surgeon General Dr. David Satcher during a media- covered groundbreaking ceremony. Allen Temple also supports an orphanage in Zimbabwe of 160 children suffering with AIDS by providing housing, medical care and supplies. The programs highlighted in this chapter are a small sample of the multitude of program services established by the Allen Temple Church in the Oakland community. It is with great expectation that the Care Advocate Program continue the historical outreach efforts that Allen Temple has provided for the past 85 years as an institution of spiritual, educational and political prominence.

Why Engage Black Churches in the Effort to Stop Elder Abuse in Nursing Homes

Allen Temple is one of the largest Black churches in Oakland and has members who reside in nursing homes that could be at risk for elder abuse. Most Black churches have a ministry that visits the "sick and shut-in" and many pastors have taken a special interest in collaborating with the Care Advocate Program to stop elder abuse. Recent literature suggests that the informal support offered by black churches plays a particularly important role in the lives of older African-Americans (Walls, 1992). Historically, black churches have been seen as a viable source of support for providing informal services to African Americans, because of the advocacy and extended kin roles they have played in the community (Poole, 1990; Taylor, Thornton and Chatters, 1987). Research reveals that elder' perceptions of black churches are strong and may contribute to the ability of the churches to serve as an important resource in enhancing minority elders use of formal services or their ability to cope with life changes (Walls, 1992).

Responding to Elder Abuse: The Care Advocate Program

As a means of responding to this problem I initiated the Care Advocate Program that educates participants on how to observe, intervene and report elder abuse if detected. The program also teaches participants methods of advocating on behalf of the senior and their families in an effort to curtail the incidence of abuse found in these settings. This is achieved through collaboration with professionals from key elder abuse prevention agencies, medical providers who have expertise on senior care and computer training utilized to access elder abuse information. Specifically it works with participants in the community and educates designated leaders of the church on elder abuse in institutional settings. The training aims to prepare participants to provide a friendly visiting service for seniors that reside in these settings and to set in motion the same service in other churches in the community. These individuals then initiate a friendly visiting service where they can detect, report and intervene on behalf of seniors and their families when elder abuse has been identified.

Because I believed the Care Advocate Program could become a model for addressing elder abuse in nursing homes, I wanted to study its implications and impact. Specifically, I administered a pre-test, conducted three classroom training sessions, four facility site visits and gave a post-test to determine the ability of participants to engage in a friendly visiting service that observes, intervenes and advocates for elderly residents and their families in a nursing home setting. This dissertation details what I learned. Specifically in the chapters to follow, I provide a literature review that documents the problem of elder abuse in an institutional setting. I present a description of the Care Advocate Program and explain how it aims to respond to these problems. Next I detail my methods, discuss my findings and their implications.

PROCEDURE FOR OBTAINING SAMPLES

Sample- Participant Trainees

Three weeks prior to the first Care Advocate Program training, Pastor Dr. J. Alfred Smith Sr. preached a sermon called "Do You Care". This sermon was given during Sunday morning communion service, which typically has the highest attendance rate, to emphasize Allen Temple's continued commitment to the care of seniors who reside in nursing and convalescent homes in our congregation. Information regarding the training was published in the weekly church bulletin on bright colored paper with a C.A.P. telephone number for interested persons to contact.

The C.A.P. training was open to members and non-members of Allen Temple from all backgrounds to encourage an unrestricted range of persons interested in advocating on behalf of seniors residing in long-term care settings to attend. The initial telephone calls came from people who wanted to ask questions about a loved one in a nursing home and gather additional information regarding the program.

When people began to arrive for the first training session, it was apparent to me that there would be two categories of people who attended. The first group included persons that came to the training to gain personal knowledge on the topic, learn how to advocate for better care of a loved one but did not wish to be apart of a research study. These individuals could choose to attend one or all of the sessions without any obligation to complete the coursework and could attend at their leisure to learn more about institutional elder abuse. In total, 23 members attended one or more trainings, but chose not to participate as care advocates.

The second category of participants that attended the C.A.P. program will be referred to as participant trainees. These trainees expressed a clear interest and agreed to complete all required training sessions, nursing home site visits and written assignments so that the required data could be collected for this research study. There were six persons from the group that consented to be participant trainees and complete 12 hours of Care Advocate Program training for three consecutive Saturdays over a three- week period of time. The participant trainees were comprised of five women and one man from varying professional backgrounds between the ages of 35-55 years of age. The trainees and I discussed the basis of this research study, goals of the program and a period of time was set aside to answer questions. Once a clear understanding of the program had been achieved, I obtained written informed consent from each trainee and emphasized confidentiality to assure their responsibility for the protection of names, study contents and any other identifying information during the course of training. The trainees understood the importance of their participation in this doctoral research study and agreed to stay in the program for the entire training process to assure accurate gathering of data. All trainees completed the entire course.

Sample- Participant Residents

Allen Temple has 23 seniors who are members of the church residing in nursing homes or similar settings. With the pastor's approval, I was given a list of these members and randomly visited each one to discuss the program and potentially obtain consents for participation in the Care Advocate Program training. Some of the seniors on the list that were visited could not speak, process information and received total patient care due to advanced illness. I methodically went down the list to identify other seniors who were able to understand and engaged in conversation regarding participation in the program.

As a result, three seniors in three separate facilities were chosen for this study.

Instruments

Four data collection tools were used as a method to gain insight and document what was learned during the Care Advocate Program training process. The four tools include a Pre-test, Facility Checklist, Observational Checklist, Post-test and Family Communication Form.

Pre-Test

A pre-test was given to gather baseline data about the trainees' knowledge and attitudes toward the elderly and institutional settings (See Appendix A).

Facility Checklist

The facility checklist is a five- page questionnaire that trainees used as a guide to observe specific areas of resident care, environmental safety and staff relations found in nursing homes that could potentially indicate signs of abuse and/or neglect (See Appendix B).

Observational Checklist

The observational checklist is an instrument that was used to evaluate the observation skills of the trainees while shadowing them for one hour during their final nursing home site visit (See Appendix C).

Facility and Observation Checklist Content

The facility and observational checklists are exactly the same. The trainee completed the facility checklist and the trainer completed the observation checklist. The facility checklist and observational checklist are designed to standardize the evaluation process of observing resident care and nursing home conditions taught during classroom training sessions. There are twelve areas of resident care and safety that include the following areas of observation:

Environment: Many times when one walks into a nursing home, there is a strong smell of urine, which could indicate that residents are not being diapered or toileted properly. The nursing home environment can often be unclean and have clutter, which may be indicative of how they treat the resident. If the facility maintenance does not clean the facility that could raise some question about how clean they keep the resident. Seniors in these settings are typically frail and vulnerable and an open door policy with no security system in place could lead to unwanted visitors. The abuse protection agency that is designated to serve seniors in a nursing home is Ombudsman. C.A.P. trainees check the environment for the state mandated Ombudsman sign that is to be posted wheelchair level in the lobby.

Visit: Trainees were educated that seniors are dying in nursing homes from dehydration and malnutrition. It was important to include what time and day trainees visited and if they did so during mealtimes. As per our discussion in the Literature Review, seniors who receive regular visits are less likely to be abused. The second component of the facility observation was to document when trainees visited and if they had the opportunity to speak with the family during the visits.

Survey: It is state mandated that all licensed nursing homes must post a recent Department of Health survey. The third component of the facility observation was for trainees to see if in fact it was posted but not bring attention to themselves if is was not.

Many times nursing home staff feels uncomfortable when you ask them for a survey because this document reveals all problems areas found by state health facility evaluators.

Relationships: Most nursing homes have a staffing shortage and poor nurse-resident ratios, which can potentially affect the relationship nurses' have with the senior. The fourth component of the facility observation was to evaluate how the nurse related to the resident by focusing on their eye contact, tone of voice and interpersonal relationships with others.

Hygiene: One of the causes of death in nursing homes is an infected bedsore, which **is** also known as decubitus. The fifth component of observation was to focus on the resident's hygiene to determine if they were well groomed, wore clean clothing and had proper oral care.

Toileting: Because nursing homes are short staffed, many seniors are not taken to the bathroom regularly, do not have their diapers consistently changed and are often left lying in their own urine and feces for extended periods of time. Another cause of death of seniors in nursing homes is urinary tract infections, which is why the sixth component of observation evaluates toileting.

Nutrition and Hydration: The seventh component of observation addresses the issue of malnutrition and dehydration, which leads to death of seniors in a nursing home. Trainees were educated to evaluate the seniors' nutritional intake and if fresh water is at the bedside. Many seniors in a nursing home are not able to feed themselves and the staff is too busy to assist them leading to malnutrition. Seniors typically have swallowing difficulties and are not offered water, which could lead to dehydration.

Safety: One of the key factors to resident neglect and abuse is their inability to reach the call light or have access to a telephone. Access to a telephone or call light is often disregarded by nursing home staff and limits the seniors' ability to call for help or notify a loved one if they are being abused or neglected. The eighth component is essential to the trainees' role as advocates to act on their behalf in placing a call to protective service agencies if abuse is suspected. It has always been my contention that if the senior could not reach a telephone to call Ombudsman, what difference did it make that it was posted in a lobby that they could not see. Safety is crucial because seniors in nursing homes are often isolated, bed bound and a fall risk.

Medications: The nurse that dispenses medication in a nursing home is typically a licensed vocational nurse who is required to provide medication and treatments to more seniors than what is humanly possible in a timely manner. The ninth component educates trainees to observe the medication regime and determine if the nurse was knowledgeable about the purpose, use and dose given to the senior. As per our literature review discussion, seniors are often given medications to keep them sedated to make them less problematic for the staff.

Therapy/Medical Care: The tenth component of the facility observation process is *designed to help* determine if the resident is receiving proper therapy and or medical care. Abuse of seniors can be observed when medical care is withheld and the physician is not properly notified. As in the case regarding Helen Love, that testified how the nurse starting hitting her, fracturing her neck and wrist and the nursing home withholding medical treatment. The code of silence and cover-up when abuse has occurred in these settings is prevalent.

Signs and Symptoms: Trainees were educated to observe for signs and symptoms of abuse and or neglect. The eleventh component focuses on evaluating whether the resident has any bruises, cuts, fractures or marks that would indicate physical or sexual abuse. This component also addresses the steps that the trainee took to notify proper authorities if abuse or neglect was suspected.

Emotional: The final component of the nursing home observation process is to determine the emotional state of the resident. Abuse may be indicative if a senior is tearful, fearful, withdrawn or flinches when approached. Trainees are educated to observe the seniors mental health status because many residents living in a nursing home suffer with dementia, Alzheimer's or memory deficits. They require a greater level of advocacy due to their mental impairment that hinders them for calling for help if they are being abused.

The results of the facility site visit observations and the areas where trainees found problems are provided in the following sections for all three facilities. Trainees reported that the first visit was comparatively more problematic than the last, which indicates the nursing staff's efforts to improve the quality of resident care and safety due to the Care Advocate Program's proactive involvement.

Post Test

The post-test provided information about what was learned as a result of the training and produced data needed to evaluate the effectiveness of the program (See Appendix A).

Family Communication Form

A communication form was given to each trainee prior to their site visits and used to provide designated family members with feedback from the trainees regarding concerns they have for the care or conditions found while visiting the Allen Temple member that agreed to participate in the C.A.P. research study (See Appendix D).

PROCEDURE

Pre-test

During the first thirty minutes of the first training day, participant trainees were given a pre-test. A section of the conference room was set apart to provide a quiet place for trainees to complete a twenty question test that was used to determine their experiences and understanding of institutional elder abuse prior to Care Advocate Program training. Each trainee was given thirty minutes to finish the pre-test and puzzled expressions on some of their faces revealed uncertainty regarding the answers. Trainees were assured that there was not a right or wrong answer during pre-testing, but rather that it was a chance to gather information needed to establish their baseline knowledge.

Training Schedule

The Care Advocate Program required trainees to attend three consecutive Saturdays of classroom training for four hours, perform two facility site visits in pairs and complete an observation site visit where they are shadowed for one hour.

Family communication form

After the last facility site visit, trainees completed a family communication form that was used to provide family members with feedback and recommendations regarding the resident.

Post Test

Trainees were given thirty minutes to complete a twenty -question post-test used to determine what was learned in the training process. The post-test, a facility checklist and family communication form was submitted upon completion of the C.A.P. training.

Dinner

Trainees were invited to a dinner to thank them for all their hard work and give them an opportunity to share their experiences. All trainees were in attendance but one who was at the hospital with his wife having a baby. Trainees stated that it was significant that a baby was born at the conclusion of the C.A.P. training. Trainees felt that it marked the birth of a new intervention that they felt so proud of. One of the highlights of their conversation focused on the sense of accomplishment they had for completing four- month training and the closeness they felt toward the senior that they advocated for. They hugged each other, exchanged telephone contact information and agreed to join me for an upcoming television show featuring the Care Advocate Program.

INTRODUCTION, RATIONALE AND BACKGROUND OF QUALITATIVE RESEARCH

Qualitative research takes an interpretive, naturalistic approach to its subject matter in which qualitative researchers study things in their natural settings, attempting to make sense of, or interpret, phenomena in terms of the meaning that people bring to them (Denzin and Lincoln, 1994). Sherman and Reid (1994) define qualitative research as "research that produces descriptive data based upon spoken or written words and observable behavior". Qualitative research broadly defined, means "any kind of research that produces findings not arrived by any means of statistical procedures or other means of quantification" (Strauss and Corbin, 1990). Qualitative research is best characterized as a family of approaches whose goal is to understand the lived experiences of persons who share time, space and culture (Frankel and Devers, 2000a).

Qualitative research begins by accepting that there is a range of different ways of making sense of the world and is concerned with discovering the meanings seen by those who are being researched and with understanding their view of the world rather than that of the researchers (Jones, 1995). Qualitative research methods have a long history in the social sciences and deserve to be an essential component in health and health services research (Pope and Mays, 1995). Recent years have seen qualitative approaches to research gain increasing prominence and acceptance in many disciplinary fields, including those that are health related (Cheek, 1996). The sensitive and appropriate uses of qualitative research are providing new insights and directions about the human condition, health and education (Frankel and Devers, 2000).

Qualitative research most often uses "purposive," rather than random, sampling

60

strategies. Given the real-world context in which most qualitative research is carried out, identifying and negotiating access to research sites and subjects are critical parts of the process (Frankel and Devers, 2000b). Purposeful sampling is the dominant strategy in qualitative research and seeks information-rich cases that can be studied in depth (Patton,1990). Before any recording and analysis can take place, the setting to be observed has to be chosen this sampling is seldom statistically based. Instead, it is likely to be purposive when the researcher deliberately samples a particular group or setting (Mays and Pope,1995).

The idea of this type of sampling is not to generalize to the whole population but to indicate common links or categories shared between the setting observed and other like it. In spite of the apparent flexibility in purposeful sampling, researchers must be aware of three types of sampling error that can arise in qualitative research. The first relates to distortions caused by insufficient breadth in sampling; the second from distortions introduced by changes over time; and the third by lack of depth in data collection at each site (Patton, 1990).

The goal of qualitative research is the development of concepts which help us to understand social phenomena in natural settings, giving due emphasis to the meanings, experiences, and views of all the participants (Pope and Mays, 1995). Qualitative research uses the natural setting as the source of data. The researcher attempts to observe, describe and interpret settings as they are, maintaining "empathetic neutrality" (Patton, 1990). According to Lincoln and Guba (1985), the most useful strategy for the naturalistic approach is maximum variation sampling which aims to capture and describe central themes or principal outcomes that cut across a great deal of participant or program variation.

Any common patterns that emerge from great variation are of particular interest and value in capturing the core experiences and central, shared aspects or impacts of a program (Patton, 1990). Qualitative research, then, is a broad approach to the study of social phenomena; its various genres are naturalistic and interpretive, and they draw on multiple methods of inquiry.

Qualitative research does not designate a specific approach. Rather it signifies development of a coalition of interests and movement toward diversity of inquiry (Mullen, 1995). As Weitzman and Miles (1995) express it, qualitative research is " a big tent," covering works labeled as explanatory or positivistic, interpretivist, and critical theorist in their approaches to understanding the social world. Marshall and Rossman (1995) explain that they use the term qualitative research as a broad umbrella: " Throughout the text we refer to qualitative research and qualitative methods as if these were one agreed–upon set that everyone understands; we intend no such implication". Therefore, considerations of ontology (being in the world) and epistemology (what is to be known) are important in relation to each miniparadigm of qualitative research. Thus, qualitative research is pragmatic, interpretive, and grounded in the lived experiences of people (Marshall and Rossman, 1999).

Qualitative researchers are intrigued with the complexity of social interactions as expressed in daily life and with the meanings the participants themselves attribute to these interactions (Marshall and Rossman, 1999). Such researchers view inquiry as leading to radical change or emancipation from oppressive social structures, either through sustained critique or through direct advocacy and action taken my the researcher, often in collaboration with participants in the study (Marshall and Rossman, 1999). In qualitative inquiry, initial curiosities for research come from real-world observations, emerging from the interplay of the researcher's direct experience, tacit theories (one's personal experience), political commitments, interests in practice, and growing scholarly interests (Marshall and Rossman, 1999).

Qualitative researchers typically rely on four methods of gathering information: a) participation in the setting, b) direct observation, c) in-depth interviewing, and d) analyzing documents and material culture. These methods form the core of qualitative inquiry- the staples of the diet (Marshall and Rossman, 1999) .The two prevailing forms of data collection techniques associated with qualitative inquiry are interviews and observations. Qualitative interviews many be used either as the primary strategy for data collection, or in conjunction with observation, document analysis, or other techniques (Bogdan and Bilken, 1982). Qualitative interviewing utilizes open-ended questions that allow for individual variations. There are three types of qualitative interviewing (Patton, 1990): 1) informal, conversational interview; 2) semi-structured interview; and 3) standardized, open-ended interviews.

An interview guide or " schedule" is a list of questions or general topics that the interviewer wants to explore during each interview. Although it is prepared to insure that basically the same information is obtained from each person, there are no predetermined responses, and in semi-structured interviews the interviewer is free to probe and explore within these predetermined inquiry areas (Lofland and Lofland, 1994). Interviewing guides ensure good use of limited interview time; they make interviewing multiple subjects more systematic and comprehensive; and they help to keep interactions focused.

In keeping with the flexible nature of qualitative research designs, interview guides can be modified over time to focus attention on areas of particular importance, or to exclude questions the researcher has found to be unproductive for the goals of research (Lofland and Lofland, 1984). Interviews have particular strengths. An interview is a useful way to get large amounts of data quickly. Combined with observations, interviews allow the researcher to understand the meanings that people hold for their everyday activities (Marshall and Rossman, 1999).

The classic form of data collection in naturalistic or field research is observation of participants in the context of a natural scene. Qualitative observation involves watching, and recording what people say and do. As it is impossible to record everything, this process is inevitably selective and relies heavily on the researcher to act as the research instrument and document the world she or he observes (Mays and Pope, 1995). Observational data are used for the purpose of description- of settings, activities, people, and meanings of what is observed from the perspective of the participants (Patton, 1990). Observation can lead to deeper understandings than interviews alone, because it provides a knowledge of the context in which events occur, and may enable the researcher to see things that participants themselves are not aware of, or that they are unwilling to discuss (Patton, 1990). Therefore it is vital that the observations are systematically recorded and analyzed, either through the traditional medium of field notes written during or immediately after the events occur or by using audio or video recording equipment (Mays and Pope, 1995).

Data analysis is the process of bringing order, structure, and interpretation to the mass of collected data. Qualitative data analysis is the search for general statements about relationships among categories of data; it builds a grounded theory (Strauss and Corbin, 1997). In qualitative studies, data collection and analysis typically go hand in hand to build coherent interpretation of the data. The researcher is guided by initial concepts and developing understandings but shifts or modifies them as she collects and analyzes the data (Marshall and Rossman, 1999). Typical analytic procedures fall into six categories: a) organizing the data; b) generating categories, themes, and patterns; c) coding the data; d) testing the emergent understandings; e) searching for alternative explanations; and f) writing the report (Marshall and Rossman, 1999). The field notes gathered during observational research are likely to be detailed, highly descriptive accounts and therefore cumbersome. As descriptions alone they cannot provide explanations. The researcher's task is to sift and decode the data to make sense of the situation, events, and interactions observed (Mays and Pope).

STUDY DESIGN AND METHOD

The Care Advocate Program (C.A.P.) data was collected between September 2002 and December 2002. The four-month collection period included three consecutive Saturdays of classroom training and four facility site visits in nursing homes where an Allen Temple senior resides. There were six trainees and three seniors or a designated representative of the senior that signed consent of participation for this doctoral research study. Prior to the first classroom training session, a pre-test was given to each trainee and after the final facility site visit, a post-test was given to each trainee. After conducting two-facility site visits, trainees completed a Facility Checklist survey that highlighted areas of patient care observed during the visitation process. During the final facility site visit, I completed a Observation checklist to determine if trainees were able to assess if quality patient care was being provided and to observe the trainees ability to effectively identify and respond to elder abuse if suspected.

The data gathered from the pre and post-test was assessed by evaluating the content of the answers and the accuracy of the responses to the survey questions provided before and after the trainees had completed the training process. The responses were analyzed to understand each trainee's level of pre and post program understanding, analyzed for similarities in the responses given by trainees working in pairs and analyzed by evaluating the responses given by all six trainees.

Observational data are used for the purpose of description- of settings, activities, people, and meanings of what is observed from the perspective of the participants (Patton, 1990). Data were collected through the use of observation notes written during and after each training session. I used observation notes to capture information being presented by representatives from protective service agencies and health care providers connected with the reactions observed from trainees to the information being presented by the panels of guests. I analyzed this data by reviewing the observation notes to understand what commonalities were shared among trainees. The notes included non-verbal communication observed from the trainees' tone of voice, facial expressions and body language. Observation notes were used to document information given during the training, questions asked by trainees during the presentations and relationships of this information to the Care Advocate Program process. Any common patterns that emerge from great variation are of particular interest and value in capturing the core experiences and central, shared aspects or impacts of a program (Patton, 1990).

The goal of qualitative research is the development of concepts which help us to understand social phenomena in natural settings, giving due emphasis to the meanings, experiences, and views of all the participants (Pope and Mays, 1995). Upon completion of the classroom training sessions, six paired trainees were assigned to visit three seniors residing in nursing homes in three separate locations. After trainees conducted two facility site visits, a facility checklist was completed and used as a data collection tool to document trends and patterns noted by two trainees evaluating the same facility. The information gathered from the facility checklist was transcribed verbatim and compared between trainees paired in the same facility and those trainees evaluating other facilities. I analyzed the data from the facility checklist by reviewing similarities in the survey responses given by trainees individually and compared the responses to the trainee that paired with them and with other trainees in different facilities.

Qualitative research begins by accepting that there is a range of different ways of making sense of the world and is concerned with discovering the meanings seen by those who are being researched and with understanding their view of the world rather than that of the researchers (Jones, 1995). During the final facility site visit, I shadowed trainees for one hour and evaluated their ability to identify patient care concerns, intervene with nursing home staff and advocate on behalf of the senior being visited. I completed an observation checklist after the final facility site was conducted to evaluate the observation skills of paired trainees, obtain feedback from the resident participating in this research study and establish the quality of care being rendered in the nursing home facility. I analyzed the data from the observation checklist by categorically documenting the results of my findings and using this information to find commonalities in the experiences of six trainees, three seniors and three facilities involved in the Care Advocate Program training.

Qualitative researchers are intrigued with the complexity of social interactions as expressed in daily life and with the meanings the participants themselves attribute to these interactions (Marshall and Rossman, 1999). The data collection tools for this research study provided me with information necessary to understand the trainees prior program knowledge, experiences with observing and interacting with nursing home residents and staff and level of knowledge received after completing the training program. At the end of the facility visits, trainees completed a communication form that provided feedback to the family. Trainees used the family communication form to give recommendations about quality of care issues observed in the facilities and to share information about the wishes of the senior being visited. The communication form was also used to update the family about the status of their loved one living in the facility and to educate family members about the options they have to enhance the seniors living conditions. The information on the Family Communication Form was completed by trainees and given to the family verbatim from the data collection tool.

Qualitative research is a broad approach to the study of social phenomena; its various genres are naturalistic and interpretive, and they draw on multiple methods of inquiry (Weitzman and Miles, 1995). Engaging in a variety of observations, evaluating pre and post-test findings and reviewing the results of survey questions analyzed the information gathered during this research study. This process provided me the opportunity to gain insight into the trends and patterns of a nursing home environment, the care received by senior residents being evaluated, the role of the trainee as an advocate in protecting seniors from suspected abuse or neglect and effective interaction with families.

ORGANIZING AND ANALYZING QUALITATIVE DATA

Organizing Data

Each trainee, facility and resident was assigned a number that was used to organize and track qualitative data obtained from the pre-test, facility checklist, observation checklist, family communication form and post-test findings. This allowed the researcher to arrange pertinent program data based on a numbering system designated on each data collection tool. The numbering system was established as follows:

Trainee:

Byron: Trainee # 1   Felicia: Trainee # 4

Erika: Trainee # 2   Helen: Trainee # 5

Lynn: Trainee # 3   Cathy: Trainee # 6

Facility:

Broadway Terrace: Facility: # 1

Rosedale Gardens: Facility: # 2

Valle Vista Place: Facility: # 3

Resident:

Susan: Resident # 1

Lillie: Resident # 2

Carolyn: Resident # 3

Tracking Qualitative Data

The following numbering system was used to track data on all collection tools:

Trainee #1   Facility #1   Resident #1

Trainee #2   Facility #1   Resident #1

Trainee #3   Facility #2   Resident #2

Trainee #4   Facility #2   Resident #2

Trainee #5   Facility #3   Resident #3

Trainee #6   Facility #3   Resident #3

Instruments:

Numbers designating the trainee that completed the instruments, the facility where the

training was conducted and the resident that was assigned to the paired trainees organized

the tools used to collect data. This allowed the researcher to have a complete view of the data collected throughout the training process for each trainee, facility and resident. The pre-test, facility checklist, observation checklist, post-test and family communication form was organized using the previously discussed numbering system. For example:

Pre-test:

Trainee #2

Facility #1

Resident #1

Facility checklist:

Trainee # 2

Facility #1

Resident #1

Observation checklist:

Trainee #2

Facility #1

Resident #1

Post-test:

Trainee #2

Facility #1

Resident#1

Family communication form:

Trainee #2

Facility #1

Resident #1

Color-coding:

Once all the instruments were collected from each trainee, they were then color-coded and placed individually in a plastic report cover to preserve the document. The tools were then placed in a three- ring notebook that was sectioned by colors to for immediate trainee identification at-a- glance. The color-coding system was as follows:

Trainee #1   Red

Trainee #2   Blue

Trainee #3   Green

Trainee #4   Orange

Trainee #5   Yellow

Trainee #6   Pink

Data Collection

Classroom Data

Classroom data were collected through the use of field notes by maintaining an observation log for each training session. My overall goal in the classroom observation was to maintain a field note journal to document elder abuse information provided by paneled guess, record the interactions between participants and panelists and capture the trainees' verbal and non-verbal responses to the information shared

Pre and Post-test Data

Pre-test data was collected from each trainee during the first classroom training session and the post-test was collected after the final facility site visit. The 20 question responses to both the pre and post-tests were copied to preserve the original document and copies were cut and pasted to a single piece of paper so that the researcher could view the data at-a-glance to determine common trends. For example: All answers given for question #1 by each trainee was placed on a single piece of paper and all answers given for question#2 was place on a single piece of paper until all twenty answers for both the pre and post- tests were compiled. The responses given by trainees on the pre and post-test survey was reported verbatim and sequenced in the previously discussed numbering system.

Facility Checklist Data

Each trainee completed a facility checklist even though they worked in pairs. The trainees used the facility checklist to document the two facility site visits that were completed without the researcher present.

Observational Checklist Data

The researcher shadowed trainees for one hour and evaluated their observation skills during the final facility site visit. The researcher documented the observation findings after each pair of trainees had completed the final visit.

Family Communication Form

The family communication form was completed after the final facility site visit and presented to the family by the researcher. The trainee shared concerns and provided feedback regarding their assigned senior to the designated family member using the family communication form.

Analyzing Classroom Data

Reviewing field notes and documenting common themes observed by the researcher analyzed classroom data. The field notes focused on capturing elder abuse information presented and the observation of trainees' emotions, non-verbal responses and interactions with panelist.

Instruments

Once the instruments were collected and organized, the data was then analyzed to determine common themes and patterns of information. The responses given by the trainees were documented verbatim from the data collection tools. The data collected was compared between trainees paired in the same facility with the same resident and then cross-compared with other trainees, residents and facilities visited. For example: analysis of data provided by Trainee #1 and #2 regarding the environmental safety hazards of Facility #1 was compared to the information other trainees had given about environmental safety hazards in their facilities to determine if there was a common trend.

Pre-test and Post-test Analysis:

Writing verbatim the responses that were provided by the trainees and then comparing the quality of answers provided achieved analysis of the pre and post-test.

Facility Checklist Analysis:

Each facility checklist was reviewed individually and then compared to the trainee that paired in the same facility. Once each facility checklist was reviewed and comparisons completed, the information was then documented verbatim. See Facility Checklist Findings.

<u>Observational Checklist Analysis:</u>

The observation checklist findings were summarized based on the overall evaluation of the trainees during the final observation visit. Analysis of trainees' observation skills was documented in the Observation Checklist Summary.

V. DISCUSSION OF DATA

The discussion of data includes three components: 1) I describe each facility visited by C.A.P. trainees. 2) I detail the prominent problems that were uncovered by the trainees at each facility and the degree that the problem was addressed highlighting the strategies trainees used; 3) Finally, I detail the facility observation checklist.

Broadway Terrace

Description

The first pair of Care Advocate Program trainees, Byron and Erika, was assigned to a ninety-nine-bed nursing home in Oakland. The Allen Temple member that resides there is, Susan, an eighty-nine year old woman who is alert, oriented and extremely jovial. She is known in the facility as the "lady who is always smiling" and uses her outgoing personality to watch nursing staff and see what is going on with the two residents sharing her room. One of her roommates was unable to speak, contracted into a fetal position and had intravenous fluids infusing in her arm. The other was a bed bound obese woman who spoke English as a second language. Susan jokingly told trainees that it was her job to make sure her roommates were safe because she was older than they and her bed was closest to the hallway door. Susan recently underwent an amputation of her left leg requiring twenty-four hour care in a nursing facility that provides her with physical and occupational therapies. I met with Susan prior to trainees' first facility site visit to introduce myself, discuss the program and obtain her signature for consent of participation.

One week after my initial visit, I brought both trainees to meet Susan and familiarize them with the facility where they would be conducting unannounced visits for training. As we entered the facility, a licensed vocational nurse seated at the first nurses station, greeted us and directed us to the far end of the building where Susan's room could be located. When we entered, she expressed delight that we were there and told everyone that we were her visitors from the church. Byron and Erika engaged in conversation with Susan, confirmed a follow-up visit and introduced themselves to her roommates. Even though the third roommate was unable to respond, she did blink her eyes to acknowledge their greeting. Trainees were educated about the characteristics of a senior that lives in these settings and about methods of understanding and communicating with a non-verbal resident because elder abuse is more likely to occur with seniors who cannot speak for themselves, have infrequent visitors and medical conditions that isolate them from the activities of the facility. As we were leaving the facility, a young woman approached us stating that she was a member of Allen Temple, had heard about the C.A.P. program and requested that trainees keep an eye on her mother who is mute. Byron and Erika talked about whether the two mute residents, who were not apart of the doctoral research study, could receive visits from a C.A.P. trainee. According to Ombudsman guidelines, trainees are considered to be mandated reporters and could anonymously report to a protective service agency if abuse were suspected. Trainees understood their role as advocates extended beyond the seniors involved in this program and reassured the young woman that they would indirectly observe for her mother's safety.

Problem observed and C.A.P. trainee response

The C.A.P. program encourages trainees to visit during mealtimes to determine whether the resident's nutritional and hydration needs are being met. Byron and Erika reported that they visited Susan during the dinner hour and her meals appeared nutritionally balanced and warm when presented. She also had fresh water at her bedside and was able to feed herself without assistance. The third roommate, however, could not eat food and was dependent on intravenous fluid to provide nourishment. While they conversed with Susan, the alarms on the intravenous fluid machine began to sound alerting them that there was a problem but no nurse came to check on it. Trainees observed that the bag that held the intravenous fluid for this mute resident was empty so they pushed the call light to summon nursing assistance. No nurse responded to the call light.

Byron reported that there was blood backing up inside the intravenous tubing and the need for nursing assistance was imperative so they went to the nurses' station to find help. When they got to the station, which is a short distance from Susan's room, they found three nurses seated directly under the call light panel with flashing lights and ringing bells sounding talking among themselves with no apparent intention of responding. One nurse seated at the station told trainees that a medication nurse would be there to hang a new I.V. bottle but a sufficient amount of time went by and no one came. The trainees went to the nurses' station again and down the corridor where they were told she was and found the medication nurse. She was apologetic and provided the necessary I.V. supplies to correct the problem.

Observation Checklist Summary

When I met the trainees at the facility, it was clear that they, the senior resident and the nursing home staff were familiar with each other and had established a rapport. For example, when I entered with the trainees, the nursing home staff got up, greeted both trainees by name, gave a brief update on how Susan was doing and thanked them for the baked goods they brought. This was not the case on the first visit. Byron and Erika knew if there was a security system in place, if the entrance to the nursing home was secured and when to expect a receptionist at the front desk. They could tell me where the Ombudsman sign was posted and the highlights of the Department of Health survey results that they reviewed on their first visit. Trainees knew the lay out of the building, where and what therapy services were provided and the printed resident recreational activities scheduled for the month.

As we walked down the hallway towards Susan's room, the staff at the second nurses' station also greeted trainees by their first name and began to update them on her progress. They told trainees how she slept that night, how much of her meals she had consumed, that there was fresh water at her bedside and her progress with physical therapy treatment. When we entered Susan's room, she was so excited to see us and told me how much she appreciated her new friends. Trainees hugged her and greeted her roommates. I told Susan that I was there to see how much her friends had learned during their last few visits when she pulled back the curtain to show us a wall of pictures of her family and friends. Susan is the mother of one of the leaders of the Black Panther Party, Bobby Hutton and she affectionately referred to him as her Bobby. It was a memorable experience listening to Susan talk about her life history. Trainees methodically pointed out areas of observation asked on the checklist while we were in the resident's room but the discussion of findings continued once we were outside the facility. I questioned trainees about resident hygiene and toileting, environmental safety, nutrition and medication regime to determine their ability to observe and evaluate specific areas of resident care. Trainees were able to give quality answers about these areas of care and provide detailed information on the facility checklist.

One of the highlights of this observation process was to see how the trainees interacted with the nursing home staff. Byron and Erika had addressed the nurses on numerous occasions about not answering resident call lights but when two of the nurses saw trainees coming down the hall, they immediately reported that call lights were not ringing and a meeting with the nursing supervisor had occurred to improve their response to resident needs. Byron is a charming gentleman with years of health care experience that was able to address the nurses in a pleasant but firm manner. He can be described as a person with charisma who has the knack for talking to people in a way that offers humor but demands results. I stood at the nurses' station listening to him talk to the nurses in a way that made them want to do better and feel appreciated for their efforts. For example: Byron addressed the nurses about the call lights. He leaned over the nurses' station and told them that he would be more than happy to be of assistance so that call lights would not continue to ring. On the next visit, they told him that a nurses meeting was held to discuss how they could be more responsive to a resident who has pushed their call light. Erika interacted with the staff in a passive and soft tone of voice, which is her nature, to express concern for what was best for Susan. She approached the nurses with nurturing quality to her voice that made them want to help her. For example: Erika genuinely explained to the nurses seated at the station that she really needed their help, how special they were for caring and how much she appreciated their time and efforts. The nurses responded immediately. Trainee had their own style of communicating their expectations of quality nursing care for Susan and other residents. Trainees made a point to compliment the staff, give them recognition with kind words and brought edible treats to show appreciation for their hard work.

Facility Checklist Findings (Problems are in bold text)

Environment

- The facility was clean, free of clutter and had no urine smell.
- There were wheelchairs, walkers and other assistive devices cluttering the hallways during evening visits.
- There was an Ombudsman sign posted in the facility entrance that was wheelchair level.
- There was limited or no storage space.
- **The facility had no security and open door access.**

Visit

- Trainees visited in the evening unannounced during the dinner meal.
- Erika documented that she had the opportunity to meet the family and discuss her visits. She further stated that the family told her how much her visits helped Susan.

Survey

- Trainees did not have to request the Department of Health survey because it was posted in the lobby and available for review.

Relationships between residents and staff

- **The nursing home staff did not respond to call lights when residents needed help.**
- The nurses' aide had seven to nine residents to care for and that used a normal tone of voice when speaking to the resident.
- **The medication nurse did not respond to the alarms sounding on a resident's intravenous machine.**
- The staff was polite, friendly and courteous when interacting with the resident.
- Staff made eye contact with the resident during their interaction and the interpersonal relationships were good.
- **The nurses seated at the station did not respond to trainees request for help of a resident when blood began to back up in the intravenous tubing.**

Hygiene

- The resident was well groomed, wore clean clothing and socks. She had her own teeth and good oral hygiene.
- The bed linen was tidy and fingernails were trimmed.
- Erika documented that the resident received a bed bath and several bottles of lotion was on her bedside table.

Toileting

- **Trainees did not observe the resident being assisted to the bathroom.**
- **The nurse aide did not know if the resident wore protective undergarments.**

- Erika stated that she had no smell of urine or body odor.

Nutrition/Hydration

- **Resident was not taken to the dining room for dinner and was able to feed herself.**
- The food was warm and there was fresh water at the bedside.

- **There was no interaction between the staff and resident during mealtime.**

Safety

- The resident was wearing an identification armband and the call light was in reach.
- The side rails on the bed were up and the telephone was also in reach.
- Susan was a recent below the knee amputee.
- She had a foot cradle and special padding on the bed.
- She did not appear concerned about her safety.

Medication

- Trainees did not observe Susan being given medication during their visits.

Therapy/Medical Care

- Trainees did not observe therapy or medical care being rendered.

Signs/Symptoms

- No injuries, abuse or restraints were observed.

Emotional

- Resident appeared happy with no mental health issues were addressed by the staff.
- Erika documented that she made many visits to the resident and each time her emotional states was happy and content.

Rosedale Gardens

Description

The second pair of Care Advocate Program trainees, Lynn and Felicia, was assigned to a sixty-bed facility that is located a short distance from a large medical center in Oakland. This facility is unique because it has won awards for providing quality nursing home care; rehabilitation services and end-of-life hospice care. The Allen Temple member that resides there, Lillie, was admitted after being discharged from the medical center for respiratory distress, shortness of breath and pneumonia. Lillie is alert, oriented and knowledgeable about her medical condition and the plan of care she is expected to receive in this nursing home. Lillie is staying in a private room and has numerous pieces of respiratory equipment available to assist her if she experiences breathing difficulties.

When I met with Lillie to discuss the C.A.P. program and obtain consent of participation, she informed me that her niece was also a member of Allen Temple and wanted to meet with me. As I left the building, I ran into her niece unexpectedly at the front door and realized that we have been working closely on senior issues at the church for years. She is the senior services coordinator of an Allen Temple senior retirement complex and was delighted to have her aunt participate in the program.

Several days after my initial visit with Lillie, I brought Lynn and Felicia to meet her. She was seated in a wheelchair with a respiratory therapist administering a nebulizer treatment. This breathing treatment aerates the lungs and creates a copious amount mist through a mask, which would have made it difficult for us to converse with her. While she was completing the treatment, trainees and I walked around the facility observing the activities of other residents, greeting the nursing staff and checking for licensing required items in the lobby. There was another Allen Temple senior, Belinda, who resides in this facility but was unable to participate in the program due to her frail condition. Belinda is in her nineties and was being monitored by an end- of- life specialty nurse from an agency that comes into the facility to provide hospice care. She had family members at her bedside round-the-clock and we had the opportunity to interact briefly with them.

The C.A.P. program educated trainees about medical conditions that affect the senior population and the signs and symptoms of illnesses commonly seen in nursing home residents. Trainees had the chance to see both a senior who would recover from her illness with proper treatment modalities being rendered and another who was transitioning into end-of-life care in the same nursing home facility.

Problem observed and C.A.P. trainee response

Lynn and Felicia came back to visit Lillie several days later during dinner time and reported that the nurse on duty left her meal sitting on the bedside table without offering it to her. Lynn being a registered nurse of thirty years expressed concern to the nurse that the resident should be offered her dinner while warm, be allowed to take a short rest and then be given her respiratory treatments. The nurse replied that she had a lot of work to do and she did not have time to be concerned about whether someone ate a warm meal. The nurse further stated that she had to do treatments when it was convenient for her and not the resident. The C.A.P. program taught trainees about how nursing home routines could potentially lead to resident neglect because of staff inflexibility and their personal frustrations in the workplace. They learned methods of advocating for the resident when routines are at the convenience of the nursing staff and not in the best interest of the senior. As a nurse, Lynn was able to assess that Lillie was not having any respiratory distress and there was no clinical reason why she should not be allowed to eat her meal.

Interestingly enough, Lillie stated that she watched the nursing routines on each shift and knew which nurses would get annoyed if she asked to eat first. Felicia stayed with Lillie while Lynn approached the nurses' station in a non-threatening manner to address the issue and the nurse was very apologetic. Lynn stated that one of the nursing staff even went out of their way to offer both trainees dinner as well. When Lynn got back to the room, Felicia told her that a nurses' aide had come into the room to remove the dinner tray and stated that it was her job to pick up the trays whether Lillie ate or not because the trays had to be taken back to the kitchen at a certain time.

The C.A.P. program educated trainees about nutritional deficits, malnutrition and dehydration, that could lead to the death of a nursing home resident from being deprived of food and water. When a senior resident eats slow or needs assistance to be fed, the nurses will take the tray of food, not offer it to the senior and often eat it themselves. Lillie was not at risk of being nutritionally deprived but a frail resident like Belinda would be if steps were not taken to address it. Trainees advocated for Lillie to receive her tray, which resulted in her meal being warmed, time allowed for her to eat and her breathing treatment given when she finished.

Observation Checklist Summary

Lynn and Felicia also met for approximately thirty minutes prior to my arrival to review the checklist that I would be using as a tool to observe them for this fourth facility site visit. The facility is small and there is a nurse's station as soon as you walk in with someone to greet you and have you sign the visitor's log. When we entered, the nurse seated at the station was pleasant and spoke to both trainees with familiarity because she was on duty the last two visits completed. Trainees reported that the front door was secure and locked after six o'clock in the evening. They were able to show me the Ombudsman sign posted in the hallway and stated that the Department of Health survey was missing even though there was a sign clearly directing the reader to where it should have been located. The facility layout is in somewhat of a horseshoe shape with only one nurses' station. Lillie's room is located to the right of the station so we had to pass physical therapy and the office of a facility social worker. The social worker came out of her office, shook our hands and offered any assistance that she may be able to render.

As we passed her office, trainees pointed out a physical therapy apparatus, wheelchairs, hoyer lifts and a large scale that was left blocking hallways, doorways, fire extinguishers and emergency exits. Trainees took the initiative to go back to the social workers office to politely address their concern and she told them that due to minimal storage space there was no place to put it. When we entered Lillie's room she reached her arms out to both trainees to give them a hug and started telling them of her day. She stated that she was tired because a woman down the hall kept screaming all night and no one would help her. When trainees asked the medication nurse about this woman, she stated that she does it all the time so they just ignore her. I walked down the hallway near this woman's room and she called out to me for help. When I asked her what kind of help she needed, she said that she was scared. Often seniors like this have dementia and need reassurance, which nursing home staff typically does not have time to provide on an individual basis.

We began reviewing aspects of resident care on the checklist by having trainees discreetly talk through the process of observing her hygiene and hydration. She was well groomed, neatly dressed, had fresh water at her bedside and wore foot protectors. Lillie mentioned that she was not able to get help going to the bathroom, decided to go alone knowing that her doctor had advised against it. She told trainees that when she pushed the call light, it took the nurses too long to come help her and did not want to have an accident. Medications were not given during this visit but trainees did engage in conversation with the medication nurse, while I observed their interaction, about Lillie's medication regime and she was very knowledgeable. She knew the kind of medication, the dose and the rationale for administering them based on Lillie's respiratory illness. No respiratory therapy treatment was given during this visit but the respiratory therapist recognized the trainees and spoke to them in a friendly manner.

Staff interactions with the trainees were a highlight in this shadowing process and it appeared that a good rapport had been established by the staff's response to their visit. The staff made a concerted effort to be cordial and helpful to the trainees. During their last visit, the staff offered trainees dinner when they were addressed about Lillie's meal being left on her bedside table. Lillie began to engage in conversation with the trainees about being able to leave the nursing home. They sought the social worker to discuss it and wrote a communication summary to Lillie's niece to provide her with feedback about moving her to a higher level of care, preferably a senior housing facility for independent living. Given Lynn's background, she had recommendations of facilities that Lillie's niece could have for future reference when it was time for discharge.

Facility Checklist Findings

Environment

- The facility was clean and had no urine smell.
- Wheelchairs, physical therapy apparatus, a large scale and a hoyer lift blocked hallways, doorways, fire extinguishers and emergency exits.
- There was a Ombudsman sign posted in the facility entrance.
- The front door was open but did have a security alarm that was locked after visiting hours.
- There was limited or no storage space.

Visit

- Trainees visited unannounced in the evening and during dinner meals.

Survey

- **Trainees documented that there was <u>no</u> Department of Health survey posted in the facility.**
- **There was a notice stating that the survey was accessible and posted in the family room. They looked for the survey in the family room and it was not there.**

Relationships between resident and staff

- The aide had seven or eight patients to care for and used a normal tone of voice when speaking to the resident.
- Lynn documented that the nurses' aide really liked Lillie and spoke to her in a soft loving tone.
- **The treatment nurse was more concerned about completing her own work than meeting the resident's needs.**
- The staff made eye contact with the resident and interacted in a respectful manner.
- Lynn reported that the staff was friendly and courteous. Felicia stated that they were polite.
- **The staff ignored a resident in the next room that was calling out for help.**

Hygiene

- The resident was well groomed, wore clean clothing and had good oral hygiene.
- The bed linen had just been changed and she wore heel protectors.
- A shower was given two to three times a week and her skin had lotion and was well hydrated.
- Lynn stated that Lillie always appeared clean and well cared for.

Toileting

- The staff did not respond to the resident's call light when she needed assistance to the bathroom.
- **Resident wears protective undergarments that are provided by her niece.**

Nutrition and Hydration

- **The nurse did not offer the resident her dinner and left it on the bedside table.**
- The resident was not taken to the dining room for meals. She opted to eat in her room.

- **The dining room staff was more concerned about picking up dinner trays at a certain time rather than if the resident had a chance to eat.**
- The resident needed help opening containers.
- **Lynn documented that no help was offered to the resident who could not open containers or cut her meat.** Lynn opened her juice, fruit cup and cut up her turkey.
- Cutting the meat was very important because the resident had a respiratory illness that could lead to aspiration if the meat was not cut in small portions.
- Lynn reported that on their last visit, the meal was warmed and looked appetizing.
- There was fresh water at the bedside and staff offered both trainees dinner on the last visit.

Safety

- The resident wore an identification armband and her call light and telephone was in reach.
- There were grab bars and a bench on rollers in the shower area.
- **Resident stated that the nurses take too long to come and help her to the bathroom so she goes without help against the recommendation of her physician.**
- She was not bed bound, the side rails were up and there was no foot cradle.
- The resident wanted to leave the nursing home and live in her own apartment.

Medication

- The resident did receive liquid and oral medication on schedule during both visits.
- The nurse identified the resident before giving the medication and she was knowledgeable about the medication being administered.

Therapy/Medical Care

- Trainees noted that the resident did receive physical therapy and her physician recommended ambulation with assistance. (See toileting)
- Trainees identified the physician caring for the resident and reported that he was contacted when the resident complained of pain on her left side. The physician responded in a timely manner and ordered hot compresses.

Signs and Symptoms

- Trainees observed that the resident had a gauze and bandage over her left ear. They inquired and found that she had irritation due to the plastic tubing from the nebulizer treatment.
- Trainees inquired about the complaints of pain on her left side. The resident and staff stated that she pulled a muscle from turning in an awkward manner.
- No abuse or neglect was observed and no restraints were used.
- The resident displayed no mental health issues and stated that she trusted her niece to make good decisions for her.

Valle Vista Place

Description

The third pair of Care Advocate Program trainees, Helen and Cathy, was assigned to a one hundred and fifty-bed nursing home in Oakland right across the street from Rosedale Gardens. Both nursing home facilities receive patients discharged from a large medical center nearby when they are not ready to go home and need to be transitioned to a less restrictive level of care for additional rehabilitation therapy services. The therapy services received in a nursing home are provided to promote body strengthening, increase endurance, and improve a patients' ability to ambulate with a steady gait in an effort to return home safely. During our initial tour, trainees and I were surprised to learn that

Valle Vista Place contracts with Alameda County Mental Health Services and has a locked psychiatric unit for clients of all ages located within the heart of the nursing home where seniors reside. The C.A.P. program educated trainees about mental health conditions that affect the senior population i.e. Alzheimer's, dementia and memory deficits but not about the psychiatric conditions found in a younger clientele. Because I am a certified psychiatric nurse, I conducted a brief overview with Helen and Cathy about the psychiatric illnesses that could potentially be observed of younger residents housed in this facility.

I did not realize until my initial visit with the third resident, Carolyn that she knew me since I was a little girl and had fond memories of attending church with my parents. As we reviewed the program and signed the consent of participation, she shared stories of raising me with both her roommates who were lying on their beds watching television. Carolyn explained that she lived in this nursing home and did not expect to ever be able to return home because she had suffered numerous falls requiring twenty-four hour care. She was primarily wheelchair bound, unable to walk without assistance and had a sign posted above the head of her bed indicating that she was on fall precautions.

This nursing home was very large, had three nurses' stations and a receptionist seated in the lobby greeting guests. When we entered the facility, I recognized the receptionist, Lawana, as a long-standing member of Allen Temple who told us that she had informed her co-workers about the C.A.P. program after reading information in the church bulletin. I introduced Lawana to the trainees, signed the visitor log and proceeded to Carolyn's room as we observed other residents, greeted nursing home staff and glanced at posted licensing information. Trainees spent time with Carolyn and both roommates talking, laughing and promised to return for a follow-up visit.

Problem observed and C.A.P. trainee response

Helen and Cathy stated that when they arrived in the evening for their first unannounced visit, a garbage can was propping open the front door security entrance and there was no receptionist or staff present. The C.A.P. program educated trainees about the need for security in a nursing home because seniors can potentially wander away from the facility due to Alzheimer's or mental impairments commonly seen in these settings. Trainees were concerned and found an employee who stated that it was left open so the staff could go outside and smoke cigarettes. As they walked down the hallway towards Carolyn's room, they observed physical therapy and janitorial equipment blocking emergency exit doors and resident doorways. They reported that the facility was extremely cluttered with wheelchairs, walkers, electrical cords and hoyer lifts left in the hallways and in front of resident rooms making it unsafe for of any resident with physical limitations.

The C.A.P. program provided trainees with information about environmental and safety hazards in a nursing home setting that could pose a risk to seniors with limited mobility. Trainees were educated, from a medical doctor who specializes in movement, to observe environmental risks and advocate for residents like Carolyn who are wheelchair bound and have restricted movement. Trainees saw the sign over Carolyn's bed indicating that she was on fall precautions and went to the nurses' station to politely inquire about the door being blocked. The nurse responded by pushing the equipment out of Carolyn's doorway into another resident room and in front of a fire extinguisher located on the wall next to an emergency exit. The nurse stated that there was no storage space and apologized for any inconvenience. Trainees went to the station to take fresh fruit and the nurses began to openly engage in conversation with them about the ongoing problems staff face when attempting to maintain resident safety precautions ordered by a physician. Carolyn told trainees that she is always concerned about falling because it is difficult to get her wheelchair around all the clutter.

When trainees visited on a Sunday afternoon, they reported that a large number of residents were seated in wheelchairs lined up against the walls and in the lobby unattended. They noticed a woman sitting in a wheelchair alone with contractures of her right hand that unexpectedly started choking on her own saliva. She began to heave, have difficulty breathing and gasping to get air. There was no staff around to observe or assist the lady so Helen stayed with her while Cathy went to find help. The C.A.P. program educated trainees about respiratory conditions common to seniors e.g. asthma, bronchitis and accidental choking that may require immediate attention to avoid aspiration. Seniors who have had a stroke often have problems managing oral secretions and should not be left unattended. Trainees were able to observe the situation quickly and get her the nursing assistance she needed to avoid respiratory distress that could have possibly lead to aspiration or pneumonia.

On the final visit made to the facility, trainees observed a young woman escorted out of the locked psychiatric unit by a staff member and left unattended in the shower room designated for senior residents. Trainees were in the dining room visiting with Carolyn and her friends when they noticed a nurse with an inordinate amount of keys hanging off her waist leaving a psychiatric patient in the nursing home area. When they discussed this with the nurses, they stated that the facility was even housing registered sex offenders who were also being left unattended. Helen and Cathy expressed concern that Carolyn and other frail vulnerable seniors could be at risk for abuse due to the mixed population of people who reside in the facility. Trainees stated that there was no resolution to this incident and that the nursing staff was also concerned about the problem of maintaining safety for the residents.

Observation Checklist Summary

Helen and Cathy are co-workers and had tested each other on checklist information prior to this final facility site visit. They were the only pair of trainees that did not have any health care experience but had worked with seniors in their church. They met me in front of the facility during the early evening hour and immediately commented on their concern about how garbage cans were used to prop the security door open that was observed on their last two visits. There was no receptionist at the front door, no nurses at the first nurses' station so we signed the visitor log and proceeded to Carolyn's room. Trainees showed me the Ombudsman sign posted in the lobby, Department of Health survey that they reviewed and a big activities calendar completed by the facility recreational therapist. They knew what kind and how often the resident was receiving physical and occupational therapy and what her functional limitations were. Carolyn was bed bound, wheelchair bound and on fall precautions. Trainees were very concerned that the side rails were up on her bed, it was pushed up against a sliding glass door that led to a busy street and she would be able to get out in case of an emergency. Trainees also pointed out how the emergency exits, fire extinguishers and hallways to the resident's rooms were blocked with wheelchairs, physical therapy and janitorial equipment.

Carolyn and her roommates greeted us as we entered the room and took turns hugging all of us. She told me that the trainees had spoken to the nurses about safety and that she would not have been able to get her wheelchair to the dining room unless they had helped her because of all the "stuff" blocking her doorway. She was afraid that she could fall and break a hip like so many of her friends who live in a nursing home. Trainees observed Carolyn's hygiene, hydration and nutrition and commented on her pretty floral dress, her new hairdo and the red fingernail polish that she was proud to show off. Nursing home residents are occasionally given a day pass to leave the facility.

Carolyn was scheduled to go on an outing with two other residents to the home of a family member where they would have a big Sunday dinner. She was very excited. Trainees checked her water pitcher on the bedside table to determine if it was fresh and it still had ice, which is an indication that the water was just provided. They watched her get her wheelchair to the door of a small bathroom and use the sink to balance herself when she needed to use the toilet, which she stated the physical therapist had taught her to do. Carolyn wanted to be as independent as possible and avoided pushing the call light for help when she could manage alone.

There was minimal interaction between the staff and Carolyn but a nurse did come to the room to push the wheelchair out of her doorway. The nurse was pleasant to Carolyn, spoke to her in a normal tone of voice and made eye contact during their interaction. Once the wheelchair was pushed aside, the nurse seemed hurried and left the room without acknowledging her roommates. No medications were given to her during their visits and trainees asked her if she had any recent injuries that could indicate abuse. None were reported. When trainees followed Carolyn to the recreation room where she and her friends would watch a movie, they sat with her and had a conversation about her care. Trainees reported and documented that she was in a cheerful mood, seems very happy and content with where she is. Trainees knew what questions to ask of the staff and resident to complete checklist information. They were observant about how the resident was being cared for and addressed the environmental safety hazards with the staff that could pose a threat to Carolyn and other residents with mobility limitations.

Facility Checklist Findings

Environment

- The facility was clean but had a strong smell of disinfectant.
- The facility had no urine smell.
- There was an Ombudsman sign posted in the facility.
- There was limited or no storage space.

Visits

- Trainees visited unannounced during the dinner meal and in the evening.

Survey

- There was a recent survey posted in the facility that was available for review.

Relationships between resident and staff

- **There was minimal interaction with the resident and the nurses' aide on the first visit.**
- Trainees stated that the Allen Temple member who worked there was very friendly and the nurses' aides were pleasant on the second visit.
- **The licensed nurses were not visible or available for residents.**

Hygiene

- The resident was well groomed and wore clean clothes.
- She had good oral hygiene and the bed linen was tidy.
- Trainees reported that she was in bed all covered up on the first visit but was up with her fingernails freshly polished for follow- up visits.

Toileting

- The resident had a small bathroom in her room that she shared with two roommates.
- Protective undergarments were worn and no urine smell was reported.

Nutrition/Hydration

- The resident was taken by wheelchair to the main dining room and she is able to feed herself.
- There was fresh water on the bedside table and her meals were hot when presented.

Safety

- **There was a trashcan that propped open the front door to the main entrance.**
- **The resident's hospital bed was pushed against a sliding glass door that led to a busy street. Trainees were concerned that when the resident was left in bed**

with the side rails up, it would further limit her mobility and ability to exit in case of an emergency.

- **Wheelchairs, walkers, electrical cords and hoyer lifts blocked doorways, hallways and emergency exits.**
- **The call light was in reach but not the telephone.**
- **The resident was wheelchair and bed bound with limited ability to ambulate alone.**
- **When the nurse was asked about a wheelchair blocking the resident's doorway, she pushed it in front of a fire extinguisher located on the wall next to an emergency exit.**
- **Trainees reported that the resident had no foot cradle but her roommate had one.**
- **There was a resident left alone in the lobby that began choking on her own saliva and no nursing home staff was available.**
- **A resident in the locked psychiatric unit was left unattended in the same area as seniors gathered in the dining room.**

Medications

- No medication was administered during the site visits.

Therapy/Medical Care

- The resident was receiving both physical and recreational therapy.
- Trainees stated she was confined to a wheelchair or bed.
- **It was unclear who the physician was for this client.**

Signs and Symptoms

- There were no signs or symptoms of abuse or neglect.
- No restraints were used and no injuries observed.

99

Emotional

- Trainees visited on a Sunday afternoon and reported that the resident was in a good mood and looking forward to an outing with a group of other residents. Helen documented that one of the resident's family members was going to prepare a meal for the group and she helped to plan the menu. Cathy stated that she was in a very good mood, laughing and talking with other residents.

VI. CONCLUSION

Trainees as effective advocates

The Care Advocate Program (C.A.P.) trainees were taught to be effective advocates. They learned to recognize the characteristics of abuse and how to identify abuse when visiting a nursing home. Trainees understood the signs and symptoms of abuse and changes in behavior that would cause concern for seniors at risk for being abused. Trainees also learned to look for physical markings and non-verbal communication a senior could display that would alert them to suspected abuse. Trainees gained knowledge and skills in observing and identifying elder abuse in a nursing home and to use this knowledge to advocate for the senior when abuse was suspected. For example: trainees understood that a senior with fingerprint bruises around their neck and blood around their gums and teeth was indicative of sexual abuse.

The C.A.P. trainees learned how to intervene when abuse was suspected and understand the process of reporting abuse to protective service agencies. Trainees were aware that a senior residing in a nursing home are commonly afraid of "telling" about the abuse because of the fear of retaliation from the perpetrator. Trainees learned how to use proactive intervention measures that reduced the risk for retaliation by engaging the nursing home staff during friendly unannounced visits. Trainees had detailed guidelines on how to report suspected abuse to protective service agencies and clearly understood the role they played to effectively advocate for the senior when abuse was suspected.

Trainees met the leaders of each protective service agency during classroom training, had an opportunity to interact with these representatives and expressed a sense of empowerment from this training to notify protective agencies when called to report elder abuse. The personal contact trainees made with protective service leaders was instrumental in navigating through the complex automated voice mail system that often causes seniors to become frustrated when attempting to call for help. During this research study, trainees did not observe elder abuse but evidence of unintentional neglect was apparent. For example: trainees observed that a senior was choking on her own saliva because she was left unattended in the facility lobby. It was a C.A.P. trainee that was able intervene and seek help in a timely manner to avoid the possibility of aspiration common to seniors.

The C.A.P. trainees learned how to effectively advocate on behalf of seniors and their families when abuse or neglect was suspected. Trainees understood that nursing homes typically have hierarchical levels of staffing that complicate the ability to report resident care concerns. The complaints of seniors are often ignored and their concerns discredited by the nursing home staff because they are overwhelmed, underpaid, overworked and under supervised. It is easier for staff to view seniors as being "old or senile" to avoid having to respond to their needs, concerns or complaints. As a result, seniors are left lying in their own waste, dying from dehydration or malnutrition and suffering infected bedsores.

Trainees learned how to advocate on the seniors behalf to alleviate social isolation, reduce the disregard for proper nutrition and promote quality resident care. This was achieved by educating trainees to make unannounced visits, approach the nursing staff in a non-threatening manner and effectively address resident care needs to bring about positive results. Trainees were instructed on how to use a C.A.P. communication form to provide feedback to the family regarding concerns for the senior resident.

Communication between the families and trainees provided a means by which trainees could address concerns regarding the senior. The communication form allowed the family member to receive information regarding their loved one that was instrumental in helping them to make health care decisions on their behalf. It also provided the family with recommendations that could be followed-up at the nursing home facility and with the staff to promote effective change for the senior visited. For example: feedback provided to the family on the communication form resulted in moving one senior to a newly built independent senior living facility.

Practices and structures that facilitated the success of trainees

Having C.A.P. trainees participate in three consecutive weeks of classroom training sessions was instrumental in their success. The classroom sessions prepared trainees for what they would experience when visiting a nursing home resident and gave them knowledge about elder abuse in a supportive classroom environment. The classroom training provided them with the opportunity to learn about elder abuse, ask questions, express concerns and engage in simulated nursing home exercises. The trainees were able to gain knowledge and skills necessary for observing, intervening and reporting elder abuse prior to entering their assigned facilities. Trainees reported that they felt better equipped to visit a nursing home, observe for elder abuse and advocate on behalf of the senior because they had a chance to practice these techniques in a classroom setting before entering the facility.

Having C.A.P. trainees interact with representatives from elder abuse reporting agencies and healthcare professionals was influential in their success. It was crucial to the structure of the Care Advocate Program that trainees receive first-hand information from highly-trained professionals in the field of elder abuse and senior care. The classroom sessions allowed trainees to learn about this difficult topic from people who have worked closely with abused seniors. The participation of these experts gave trainees a chance to not only gain insight into the problem of elder abuse but to also have one-on-one discussions with persons that they would interact with if abuse needed to be reported. For example: trainees listened to the presentation of a Lieutenant with the elder abuse division of the police department who had personally witnessed abuse against seniors and gave trainees his direct telephone number to contact him if needed.

Successfully training volunteers in the community

The Care Advocate Program has the capacity to reach varying levels of educational venues for persons interested in learning about elder abuse in nursing homes, strategies to intervene when abuse is suspected and methods to advocate on behalf of seniors and their families. It has been successfully taught to church volunteers, community leaders and Master's in Gerontology students that have adopted the C.A.P. program to reach seniors living in long-term care settings. It was my goal to create a program that provides learning flexibility to reach a wide-range of individuals and groups that can operationally teach this advocacy model in any setting. A curriculum has been developed to expand the use of this program in an effort to train a broad spectrum of individuals interested in curtailing the incidence of abuse against seniors residing in institutional settings (see Appendix E).

NEXT STEPS

It is my goal to start a non-profit organization, The Care Advocate Program, with a toll-free number that people can trust to access services for assistance. A C.A.P. logo, brochures and fliers are being created and will be distributed throughout the Oakland community to bring attention to the problem of nursing home abuse with program contact information for C.A.P. trainings. It has been my experience that people who have learned about the program through media efforts also lead to the success of capturing interested people who are willing to volunteer their time and effort for visiting nursing home settings.

The Post newspaper featured an article about the Care Advocate Program that was distributed in Oakland, Berkeley, Richmond, San Francisco and the Tri-Valley areas. It was also printed in Spanish and featured in the newspaper called the El Mundo. As a result, I have been inundated with telephone calls from people who want to participate in the training to learn how to become advocates. I have received requests from churches that want to set-up trainings for people who are designated by the pastor to perform outreach to senior members of the church living in nursing homes that and call from seniors themselves who would like to have advocates visit them.

This front-page article in the Post newspaper has given the C.A.P. program exposure to the community and opened the floodgates of interested individuals who express a desire to become advocates. I have listened to callers share their personal stories of abuse that they or someone they know has suffered and calls from people who work in nursing homes who have witnessed abuse first-hand. The owner of the newspaper has offered to print follow-up articles about C.A.P. in an effort to assist in facilitating the possibilities of identifying additional people who can implement the program and continue exposure of the program goals.

I have made arrangements to set up trainings at Allen Temple church located in East Oakland, Beth Eden church located in West Oakland and Progressive church located in the North Oakland/Berkeley areas for people who want to participate in the C.A.P. program. The trainings held at these three churches covers three large geographic areas that are close to public transportation to accommodate interested participants. I will also conduct trainings in the evenings and Saturdays to capture a wide range of individuals who work during the week but are interested and wish to participate in sessions that accommodate their work schedules.

I have accepted the opportunity to train intergenerational groups of participants from the community, churches and schools that want to learn more about advocating on behalf of seniors at risk for abuse and neglect who reside in a nursing home. The C.A.P. training is easy to understand, uncomplicated to follow and a basic process of friendly visiting for advocates who are knowledgeable about reporting abuse if suspected. People who want to participate in the program will learn how to be effective advocates in curtailing the incidence of abuse and potentially improve the quality of life for seniors residing there by establishing positive interpersonal relationships with the nursing home staff.

Collaborating with Allen Temple church has open doors of opportunity to reach and be recognized by families as an elder care consultant. Families in the church community have members living or may potentially live in a nursing home. As a result of this church exposure, family members have contacted me and invited me into the privacy of their homes to seek my advice, assist them with making decisions for their aging loved ones and open communication with other family members who may be having difficulty discussing these topics. Many families are dealing with the experience of having a senior family member whose health is declining and may require a higher level of nursing care than what can be achieved at home. The role of facilitating discussion among concerned family members has resulted in the ability of families to engage in dialogue on health care issues and make decisions that best address the needs of the senior involved.

I am now meeting with families to discuss current medical conditions, medications being prescribed, treatments that are being suggested, the possibility of nursing home placement and end of life issues that have become too difficult to address and is now a cause for family concerns. For example: I was recently invited into the home of three adult siblings that could not make a decision about what was best for their seventy-six year old father who had recently been diagnosed with a terminal condition. We were all seated at the formal dining room table with an array of educational materials that I brought providing information that addresses questions about senior services available to them. Along with discussing his medical condition, the challenges of navigating through an HMO system for medical care and physician recommended chemotherapy treatments, we also discussed issues such as having a durable power of attorney, advanced directives, hospice and nursing home care.

The family stated that they were most appreciative for this level of counseling in the privacy of their homes and kept me informed until their father's passing. Being invited into the home of families concerned about their senior loved one brought me great joy and a new outlook on achieving the broader goals of lessening the prevalence of abuse by providing C.A.P. training to families prior to a nursing home placement. This experience has shed a new light on the role of reducing the incidence of abuse by providing C.A.P. training to family members prior to the placement of a senior in these settings. The more education about senior care and services that families have can improve the facilities where quality of care is received.

There are some good nursing homes just has bad ones. It is a challenge for family members to ensure their loved one is not abused or neglected when difficult decisions to place them in a facility are necessary. The Care Advocate Program is the catalyst by which churches and interested people in the community can join the effort to protect residents who find themselves in a nursing home environment that often neglects and abuses vulnerable people who depend on them for quality care.

APPENDIX A: PRE/POST TEST

Pre and Post Tests

Volunteer Identification Code:

1. Have you ever visited a nursing home?

2. Have you ever lived in a nursing home?

3. Name the kind of places where the elderly reside when they are unable to live at home.

4. What is an institutional setting for the elderly?

5. Is elder abuse found in institutional settings?

6. Who are the typical abusers in an institutional setting?

7. Name three kind of abuses found in an institutional setting?

8. Would you report elder abuse if you had reason to believe it occurred?

9. Who would you report this abuse to?

10. Would you be interested in participating in a program that prevents abuse of the elderly in an institutional setting?

11. List three kind of facilities considered an institutional setting for the elderly.

12. Describe the characteristics of an institutional setting for the elderly.

13. Describe the characteristics of an elderly person in an institutional setting.

14. What is the definition of institutional elder abuse?

15. Name seven kinds of abuses found in an institutional setting.

16. List three reporting agencies designed to protect the elderly from abuse.

17. Define the term " fear of retaliation".

18. Explain how you would identify elder abuse.

19. Explain what steps you would take to intervene on behalf of an elderly resident when abuse is identified.

20. Describe methods that can be used to advocate and empower residents and their families to prevent elder abuse in an institutional setting.

APPENDIX B: FACILITY CHECKLIST

Facility Checklist

Environment

| 1. Was the facility clean? | Yes | No |

| 2. Was the facility free of clutter? | Yes | No |

| 3. Did the facility have a urine smell? | Yes | No |

4. Was an Ombudsman sign posted in the facility entrance at wheelchair level?
   Yes   No

5. Did the facility have open door access or were the doors secured?   Yes   No

Additional Comments:

Visit

1. What time did you visit? Morning   Noon   Night   Evening

2. What day did you visit? Mon. Tues. Wed. Thurs. Fri. Sat. Sun.

3. Was your visit unannounced?   Yes   No

4. Was your visit during a mealtime? Breakfast Lunch Dinner Snack

5. Did you speak with the family about your visit? Yes   No

Additional Comments:

Survey

1. Was there a recent survey posted at the facility?   Yes   No

2. Did you ask for the survey and review it?   Yes   No

3. Who did you ask and how long did it take them to provide it to you?
   Administrator   Nurse   Staff   Other
   Length of time: 15 minutes   30 minutes   45 minutes   60 minutes   Longer

4. Was there an incident when you requested the survey?   Yes   No

Additional Comments:

Relationships

1. What was the nurse aide relationship with the resident? Excellent   Good   Fair   Poor

2. How many residents did the nurse aide care for that day? 1-3   4-6   7-9   10-12 more

3. What tone of voice did the staff use when speaking to a resident?
   Loud   Soft   Normal   Rude

4. Did the staff make eye contact with the resident during their interaction?   Yes   No

5. Was the staff polite, friendly, and courteous when interacting with the resident?

6. What were the interpersonal relationships like between 1) staff and staff, 2) families and staff, 3) trainees and staff?   Excellent   Fair   Good   Poor

Additional Comments:

Hygiene

1. Was the resident well groomed?   Yes   No

2. Was the resident wearing clean clothing? Yes   No

3. Was the resident's hair clean and combed? Yes No

4. Were clean socks worn? Yes No

5. Did the resident have good oral hygiene? Yes   No

6. Was the resident wearing dentures and were they secure and clean? Yes   No

7. Did the resident have clean and trimmed toe and fingernails?   Yes   No

8. Were the linen and bed coverings clean and tidy?   Yes   No

9. How often did the resident receive a shower, bath, or bed bath?
   Daily   Weekly   Monthly   Not at all

10. Was lotion or skin protector applied? Yes   No

Additional Comments:

Toileting

1. Was the resident assisted to the bathroom regularly?   Yes   No

2. Did the resident have a Foley catheter?   Yes   No

3. Did the resident wear protective undergarments?   Yes   No

4. Was the resident incontinent of urine and stool? How often were they cleaned?
   Yes   No

Additional Comments:

Nutrition/ Hydration

1. Was the resident taken to the dining area for meals?   Yes   No

2. Was the resident able to feed him or herself?   Yes   No

3. If not, was food offered?   Yes   No

4. Was the food hot, warm or cold?   Hot   Warm   Cold

5. Was fresh water at the bedside?   Yes   No

6. What interaction occurred between staff and resident during feeding?
   Excellent   Good   Fair   Poor

Additional Comments:

Safety

1. Was the resident wearing an identification armband?   Yes   No

2. Was the call light in reach?   Yes   No

3. Were the side rails up?   Yes   No

4. Were there grab bars or skid protectors in the bath or shower areas?   Yes   No

5. Did the resident have on foot protectors?   Yes   No

6. Was there a telephone in the room and was it in reach?   Yes   No

7. Was the resident bed bound?   Yes   No

8. Was the resident turned every two hours?　Yes　No

9. Was there a foot cradle at the end of the bed to lift the sheets?　Yes　No

10. Did the resident appear fearful or concerned about safety?　Yes　No

Additional Comments:

Medication

1. Was the resident given medication?　Yes　No

2. Was it given in liquid form or did the pills require crushing?　Yes　No

3. Was the medication placed in the resident's mouth or in a feeding tube?　Yes　No

4. Was the nurse knowledgeable about the medication?　Yes　No

5. Was the medication given according to scheduled times?　Yes　No

6. Did the medication nurse identify the resident prior to giving medication?　Yes　No

7. Was the medication nurse familiar with the medication purpose, use and dose?
   Yes　No

Therapy/Medical Care

1. Is the resident involved in therapeutic activities e.g. occupational, physical, speech or recreational activities?　Yes　No
a.　Physical　b.　Occupational　c.　Recreational　d.　Speech therapy

2. Was the resident able to walk alone or with assistance of therapy staff?
   a. Alone　b. Assistance

3. Do you know the name of the physician caring for the resident?　Yes　No

4. If the resident required the assistance of a physician, was medical treatment rendered in a timely manner?　Yes　No

Signs/Symptoms

1. Did you observe and note any injuries, bruises, cuts or marks on the resident?
   Yes   No

2. Did you observe and note any sprains, strains, or fractures. Were casts or bandages used that would imply injury? Yes   No
3. Were restraints used on the resident?   Did they appear to cause injury?
   Yes   No   Yes   No

4. If abuse was detected, did you advocate on behalf of the resident?   Yes   No

5. Was a reporting agency contacted?   Yes   No

6. Which reporting agency did you contact and why?
   a. Ombudsman   b. Adult Protective Services   c. Dept. of Health and Human Services

7. Did you speak with the family regarding your concerns?   Yes   No

8. Did the provider have systems in place to detect and prevent abuse? What are they?
   Yes   No

Additional Comments:

Emotional

1. What was the resident's emotional state e.g. crying, tearful, happy, sad, content?

2. Were mental health issues addressed by the facility staff? Yes   No

Additional comments:

APPENDIX C: OBSERVATION CHECKLIST

Observation Checklist

Environment

1. Trainee observed facility cleanliness. Excellent   Fair   Good   Poor

2. Trainee observed facility clutter. Excellent   Fair   Good   Poor

3. Trainee observed if the facility had a urine smell. Excellent   Fair   Good   Poor

4. Trainee observed if the facility had an Ombudsman sign. Excellent   Fair Good Poor

5. Trainee observed door access and security.   Excellent   Fair   Good   Poor

Additional Comments:

Visit

1. Trainee visited: Morning   Noon   Night   Evening

2. Trainee visited: Monday Tuesday Wednesday Thursday Friday Saturday Sunday

3. Trainee's visit was unannounced.   Yes   No

4. Trainee's visit was during a mealtime. Breakfast   Lunch   Dinner   Snack

5. Trainee spoke with a family member regarding the visit.   Yes   No

Additional Comments:

Survey

1. Trainee checked for a recent survey posted in the facility. Yes No

3. Trainee asked for the survey from: Administrator Nurse Staff Other Length of time: 15 minutes 30 minutes 45 minutes 60 minutes Longer

4. Trainee experienced an incident when the survey was requested. Yes No See Comments

Additional Comments:

Relationships

1. Trainee assessed the nurse aide relationship with the resident. Yes No

2. Trainee assessed the nurse aide and resident ratio. Yes No

3. Trainee assessed the tone of voice used by staff when speaking to residents. Yes No

4. Trainee assessed the level of eye contact between staff and resident. Yes No

5. Trainee assessed whether staff was polite, friendly and courteous to residents. Yes No

6. Trainee observed and documented relationships between staff and staff, families and staff, trainees and staff using a scale of: Excellent Fair Good Poor

Additional Comments:

Hygiene

1. Trainee assessed the resident's grooming. Yes No

2. Trainee assessed the cleanliness of the resident's clothing. Yes No

3. Trainee assessed whether the resident's hair was clean and combed.   Yes   No

4. Trainee observed whether the resident was wearing clean socks.   Yes   No

5. Trainee assessed the resident's oral hygiene.   Yes   No

6. Trainee assessed if the resident was wearing dentures and if they were clean and secure.   Yes   No

7. Trainee assessed if the resident's toe and fingernails were clean and trimmed. Yes   No

8. Trainee observed whether the linen and bed coverings were clean and tidy. Yes No

9. Trainee determined how often the resident received a shower, bath or bed bath. Yes No

10. Trainee determined if lotion or skin protector was applied.   Yes   No

Additional Comments:

Toileting

1. Trainee assessed the frequency of bathroom assistance. Yes   No

2. Trainee determined if the resident had a Foley catheter. Yes   No

3. Trainee assessed if the resident wore protective undergarments Yes   No

4. Trainee determined if the resident was incontinent of urine and stool and how often they were cleaned.   Yes No

Additional Comments:

Nutrition/ Hydration

1. Trainee determined if the resident was taken to the dining room for meals. Yes   No

2. Trainee assessed if the resident was able to feed him or herself.   Yes   No

3. Trainee observed if food was offered to the resident.   Yes   No

4. Trainee assessed if the food was hot or cold. Yes   No

5. Trainee observed if fresh water was at the resident's bedside. Yes   No

6. Trainee observed staff and resident interactions during a feeding.   Yes No

Additional Comments:

Safety

1. Trainee observed if the resident was wearing an identification armband. Yes   No

2. Trainee observed if the resident had a call light in reach.   Yes No

3. Trainee observed if the side rails were up.   Yes   No

4. Trainee observed if grab bars and skid protectors were in the bath or shower areas.
   Yes   No

5. Trainee observed if the resident was wearing foot protectors.   Yes   No

6. Trainee observed if a telephone was in the resident's room and within the residents
   reach.   Yes No

7. Trainee observed whether the resident was bed bound.   Yes   No

8. Trainee determined whether the resident was turned every two hours.   Yes No

9. Trainee observed if a foot cradle was used to lift the sheets.   Yes No

10. Trainee assessed if the resident appeared fearful or concerned about safety. Yes No

119

Additional Comments:

Medication

1. Trainee observed if the resident was given any medication.   Yes   No

2. Trainee observed if the medication had to be crushed or given in liquid form. Yes   No

3. Trainee observed if the medication placed in the resident's mouth or in a feeding tube.
   Yes   No

4. Trainee assessed whether the nurse was knowledgeable about the medication. Yes No

5. Trainee assessed if the medication was given according to scheduled times. Yes   No

6. Trainee observed if the nurse identified the resident prior to giving a medication.
   Yes   No

7. Trainee assessed if the nurse was familiar with the medication purpose, use and dose.
   Yes   No

Therapy/ Medical Care

1. Trainee assessed if the resident is involved in therapeutic activities. Yes   No
   a. physical   b. occupational   c. recreational   d. speech therapy

2. Trainee observed if the resident was able to walk alone or if they required the
   assistance of therapy staff.   Yes   No

3. Trainee obtained the name of the physician caring for the resident.   Yes   No

4. Trainee determined if medical assistance was rendered in a timely manner. Yes   No

Signs/Symptoms

1. Trainee observed and noted injuries, bruises, cuts or marks on the resident.   Yes   No

2. Trainee noted sprains, strains, and fractures by observing casts and bandages that
   would imply injury. Yes   No

3. Trainee observed the use of restraints and if they caused injury.   Yes   No

4. Trainee advocated on behalf of the resident when abuse was detected.   Yes   No

5. Trainee contacted a reporting agency.   Yes   No

6. Trainee identified which reporting agency was contacted and why.   Yes   No
7. Trainee spoke with the family regarding their concerns.   Yes   No

8. Trainee assessed and documented what systems the provider had in place to detect and prevent abuse.   Yes   No

Additional Comments:

Emotional

1. Trainee assessed the resident's emotional state.   Yes   No

2. Trainees determined if the facility staff addressed mental health issues.   Yes   No

Additional Comments:

APPENDIX D: FAMILY COMMUNICATION FORM

Family Communication Form

Resident:

Trainee:

Facility:

Comments:

_____

_____

_____

_____

_____

_____

_____

_____

_____

_____

_____

_____

APPENDIX E: CURRICULUM

Activity I: Protective Service Agencies; Recognizing and Reporting Elder Abuse

Overview

Through pre-testing, videotape viewing and panel discussions, this activity leads participants to understand the process for reporting elder abuse to protective service agencies.

Time: 4 hours or 4 separate 45- minute activities

Materials: Pre-test, videotape, handouts, brochures, flip charts

Setting: Conference room

Panel: Adult Protective Services, Ombudsman, California Advocates for Nursing Home Reform, Alameda County District Attorney's Office and City of Oakland Police Department.

Procedure

Part A: What do trainees know about elder abuse prior to training? (30 minutes)

1.   Administer a pre-test of the participants' knowledge of elder abuse (see Appendix A) at the beginning of this classroom session and allow thirty minutes to complete the pre-test.

2.   Encourage trainees to engage in dialogue about the information asked on the pre-test and document their responses on a flip chart.

3.   Review the responses given by trainees on the flip chart and discuss the findings. The information that you want to point out to trainees as a result of this activity include:

- What is an institutional setting for the elderly?
- Who are the typical abusers in an institutional setting?

- What kinds of abuses are found in an institutional setting?
- What are the signs and symptoms of abuse?
- What agency would trainees report abuse to?

Part B: What does elder abuse in a nursing home look like? (25 minutes)

1. Show videotape from a Channel 2 television special news report on Nursing Home Abuse in the Bay Area featuring reporters Dennis Richmond and Leslie Griffith. A copy of the videotape can be obtained by contacting MEL media at 510 815-1565. The cost of the videotape is $15.

2. Allow trainees an opportunity to express their feelings, concerns and provide feedback regarding the information on the videotape. The following questions can structure this discussion:

- What feelings did you experience when viewing the videotape?
- What concerns do you have about the information on the videotape?
- Do you know someone who has experienced what was shown on the videotape?
- (Most of the trainees shed tears during the videotape). Can you share your personal reaction to the videotape with the group?
- Would you report abuse if you suspected it?

3. Use a flip chart to capture and bullet highlights of this discussion. The following information documented from this discussion include:

- Trainees' expression of feelings of fear, anxiety and uncertainty related to the abuse of elderly persons seen on the videotape.
- Seniors expression of hopelessness and helplessness when faced with abuse in a nursing home as shown in the videotape.
- Trainees' observations of abuse and neglect seen on the videotape.

- Use the flip chart to write questions that trainees have about the videotape.

Part C: What is the role of protective service agencies and how would trainees report elder abuse? (30 minutes for each presenter with 15 minutes for questions).

1. Allow each panelist thirty-minutes to share descriptive information about the characteristics of elder abuse and proper procedures for notifying designated protective service agencies.

- Ombudsman- the agency that responds to reports of abuse use in a nursing home setting.
- Adult Protective Services- the agency that responds to reports of abuse in someone's private home.
- District Attorneys' office- the agency that initiates legal prosecution of someone who has or is suspected of abusing a senior.
- Police Department- the Elder Abuse Division that responds to allegations of abuse.
- C.A.N.H.R.- the agency that promotes legislative processes designed to protect seniors from abuse.

2. Explain techniques that will ensure resident safety to avoid placing them at risk for further abuse.

- Visit the nursing home unannounced
- Visit the nursing home during mealtimes
- Observe the routine of the nursing home staff
- Engage in friendly conversation with the nursing staff
- Acknowledge the staff with baked goods and/or flowers

- Allow the senior an opportunity to express their concerns in a non-threatening manner.

- Interact with the family and keep the family informed of any concerns.

- Place the telephone and call light within reach of the senior in case help is needed.

3. Provide trainees with brochures, handouts and contact numbers of the protective service agencies that can be contacted if abuse or neglect is suspected.

- Ombudsman- 510 638-6878

- Adult Protective Services- 510 567-6894 or 1-866- CallAPS

- District Attorney's office- 510 569-9281

- Police Department

- California Assn. For Nursing Home Reform /C.A.N.H.R.- 1-800-474-1116

4. Provide a question-answer period for trainees to respond to the information given and ask questions of the panelists.

5. Facilitate the discussion to ensure the information is directly related to the Care Advocate Program goals.

- The facilitators will emphasis that C.A.P. trainee should not take a clipboard or any writing materials into the nursing home.
- The facilitators will emphasis that C.A.P. trainees not allow the esthetic appearance of the nursing home to hinder their ability to identify abuse.
- The facilitators will emphasis that C.A.P. trainees will experience unusual smells and sounds in a nursing home setting.

- The facilitators will emphasis that C.A.P. trainees will observe seniors with a fear of retaliation that may prevent them from "telling of the abuse".
- The facilitators will emphasis that C.A.P. trainees are friendly visitors and should never place the senior at risk by approaching an abusive employee directly.
- The facilitators will emphasis that families and elder abuse protective service agencies depend on them to report suspected abuse, which can be done anonymously.
- Use a flipchart to capture the highlights of the discussion.

Part D: Going Further

The goal of the first training session is to educate trainees about elder abuse in nursing homes and introduce them to representatives from elder abuse reporting agencies that they will contact. The following techniques for encouraging 1:1 interaction with protective service agencies include:

- Provide great food, drinks and space for trainees to interact personally with representatives of elder abuse reporting agencies.
- Encourage trainees to establish a rapport and build collaborations with representatives who will assist them when abuse or neglect is suspected.
- Give trainees a chance to ask questions on a 1:1 basis and provide personal telephone numbers of reporting agency representatives.

Activity II: Characteristics of Elder Abuse

Overview

Through panel discussions with a team of physicians and a nutritionist, trainees will be educated about the physical, sexual, emotional and nutritional effects of elder abuse that seniors could suffer in an institutional setting.

Time: 4 hours or 4 separate 45- minute

activities Materials: Brochures, handouts, flip

charts Setting: Conference room

Panel: Internist, Obstetrician/Gynecologist, Physiatrist, Nutritionist

Procedure

Part A: What do trainees know about physical, sexual and nutritional abuse that a

senior may suffer in an institutional setting? (30 minutes for each presenter and 15

minutes for questions).

1.   Allow each panelist thirty minutes to provide pertinent information regarding

the signs and symptoms of abuse from a medical perspective.

2.   Review the kinds of signs and symptoms that identify physical and sexual abuse

by using a flip chart to highlight the information shared.

- Bruises, black eyes, welts, lacerations, rope marks, imprint injuries
- Fractures
- Open wounds, cuts, punctures
- Sprains or dislocations
- Unexplained venereal disease or genital infections
- Unexplained vaginal or anal bleeding
- Bruises around the breast or genital area

3.   Open up the discussion with a question and answer period to assure that trainees

can recognize indicators of abuse and neglect.

4. Facilitate the discussion to ensure that the information is directly related to the Care Advocate Program goals.

- C.A.P. trainees will not touch or examine a senior for abuse.
- C.A.P. trainees will observe for physical markings indicative of abuse in a discreet manner.
- C.A.P. trainees will look at a senior's neck for bruises and their mouth for blood indicative of sexual abuse.
- C.A.P. trainees will listen carefully to the senior when they discuss nursing care and observe for reactions of fear when a nurse enters the room.
- C.A.P. trainees will report suspected abuse to protective service agencies and can do so anonymously.

5. Use a flip chart to capture the highlights of the discussion.

Part B: Going Further

The goal of the second training session was to educate trainees about the physical, sexual, emotional and nutritional effects of elder abuse that seniors could suffer in an institutional setting. The technique used to allow trainees a opportunity to interact with panelist include:

- Provide great food, drinks and space for trainees to interact personally with paneled health care professionals.
- Encourage trainees to establish a rapport and build collaborations with the physicians and nutritionist that can assist them with recognizing signs and symptoms of abuse and neglect that could be observed when visiting a nursing home.
- Give trainees an opportunity to interact on a 1:1 basis and share
- telephone numbers of healthcare providers who have agreed to be a clinical resource for trainees.

Activity III: Preparing to Visit a Nursing Home

Overview

Through reviewing the Care Advocate Program training manual, engaging in simulated

nursing home exercises and using a computer lab, trainees will gain access and have

increased understanding of pertinent elder abuse information.

Time: 4 hours or 4 separate 45-minute activities

Materials: Training manual, flip chart, assignment sheets

Setting: Conference room and computer lab

Procedure

Part A: How does the trainee use the C.A.P. training manual as a reference guide? (45

minutes)

1.   Use the training manual as a refresher course for trainees to review information

presented by the paneled guests in the first two classroom sessions. Sit is a circular

fashion and methodically review the training manual for the first thirty minutes of the

session.

- Discuss what institutional abuse is and methods to identify abuse.
- Review the signs and symptoms of elder abuse.
- Review the process of reporting elder abuse to protective service agencies.
- Review methods of advocating on behalf of the resident and their families if
  abuse or neglect is suspected.
- Review and provide copies of the Family Communication Form. This form is
  completed after the last facility site visit. Trainees completed the family
  communication form to provide family members with feedback and
  recommendations regarding the resident.
- Discuss methods of maintaining resident safety.

- Review the survey process conducted by a regulatory agency.

2. Allow trainees an opportunity to give personal testimonies about the impact the Care Advocate Program has had on them. Allow trainees an opportunity to candidly expressing their feelings, fears and concerns related to learning about the abuse and neglect of seniors in nursing homes.

4. Give trainees an opportunity to engage in a question and answer period to ensure understanding and clarification of C.A.P. program information is clear.

Part B: What is it like to visit a nursing home? (45 minutes)

1. Set-up the conference room to look like a nursing home:

   a. Simulate a lobby and reception area where trainees would be expected to sign in prior to entering the nursing home.
   b. Set-up nursing stations (at least two) where nurses gather and call lights are placed.
   c. Set-up a patient room that includes a bed with side rails, a side table next to the bed, a bed table that is used to place meal trays on and other beds for another resident living in the same room.
   d. Set-up a survey, Ombudsman sign and activity schedule typically seen in a nursing home foyer or hallway.
   e. Set-up an occupational, physical, speech, recreational therapy room.
   f. Set-up a dining room area/simulated meals in the patient room.

2. Allow trainees to participate in role-playing in a simulated nursing home setting.

   - Role play a nurse
   - Role play a senior/ an abused senior

- Role play a family member
- Role play the support staff
- Role play the survey process

3. Review focused role-playing activities to prepare them to:

- Ask the right questions
- Interact positively with nursing home staff
- Identify signs and symptoms of abuse
- Document pertinent facts
- Consider resident safety
- Advocate on behalf of the senior and their family
- Report suspected abuse or neglect to protective service agencies

4.Give trainees simulated nursing home activities that can prepare them for their facility visits and increase familiarity with the site visiting process.

- Evaluate the physical layout of the nursing home i.e. secure doors, the presence or lack of security.
- Evaluate the evidence of clutter, side rails and call lights.
- Evaluate the presence of identification armbands.
- Evaluate nurse-patient staffing ratios.
- Evaluate if the food is warm and if there is fresh water,
- Evaluate unusual smells and cleanliness.
- Evaluate appropriate clothing worn by the senior.
- Evaluate if restraints are being used.
- Evaluate nurse-patients interactions.

5. Encourage trainees to role-play as the visitor entering the nursing home and the role of the senior being visited.

6. Give trainees time to engage in a question and answer period for discussion.

Part C: What is the survey process and how can the survey results be accessed using the Internet? (45 minutes)

1. Secure a computer lab equipped with high- speed Internet capability.

2. Educate trainees about the survey process conducted annually on all licensed nursing homes by the State of California Department of Health Services' Licensing Division (D.H.S.).

3. Teach trainees how to use the computer lab to access the Internet for information regarding nursing homes, licensing survey results, elder abuse prevention and educational resources from the D.H.S. web site.

- http://www.aoa.dhhs.gov.
- www.aoa.dhhs/abuse/report.htm.
- http://www.aoa.dhhs.gov/factsheets/ombudsman.html.
- www.elderabuselaw.com.
- http://www.hhs.gov/news.
- www.medicare.gov/nursing/home.asp
- NCEA@NASUA.ORG.
- http://senior-site.com/nursing/abuses.html.

4. Educate trainees about the procedure used to conduct annual nursing home surveys, the role of health facility evaluators, and reviewing licensing survey reports that document quality care deficiencies found during this compliance process.

   a. Health facility evaluators from the Department of Health and Human Services for the State of California are typically registered nurses with advanced training that enter a nursing home when a complaint is filed.

   b. Health facility evaluators enter the nursing homes when an annual survey is conducted to initiate or renew facility licensure.

   c. Review an actual survey that has been completed by accessing the website (b).

5. Provide trainees with information on where to find the survey when conducting facility site visits and how to use it as a guide to identify problems in the nursing home.

   a. The survey is usually in the lobby of the nursing home.

   b. The survey may be locked in a glass wall cabinet that the trainee should request from the nurses station.

6. Give trainees time to engage in a question and answer period for discussion. Encourage trainees to peruse the Internet to learn more about elder abuse. The following topics can be accessed on the Internet to provide more information including:

   - Nursing home abuse
   - Nurses that abuse
   - Elder abuse
   - Institutional elder abuse
   - State citations on nursing homes
   - Elder mistreatment

7. Give trainees assignments for their facility site visits and provide all resource materials.

134

BIBLIOGRAPHY

ABC News. *Catching Nursing Home Abuse on Tape*: 'GrannyCams'. 7 May, 2001.Retrieved online at:

http://abcnews.go.com/sections/GMA/GoodMor/GMA010215_nursing_home_cameras.htm.

Administration on Aging, U.S. Department of Health and Human Services. Retrieved online at: http://www.aoa.dhhs.gov.

Administration on Aging, Long Term Care Ombudsman. Retrieved online at: www.aoa.dhhs/abuse/report.htm.

Administration on Aging, The Long Term Ombudsman Program. Retrieved online at: http://www.aoa.dhhs.gov/factsheets/ombudsman.html.

Adult Protective Services. Retrieved online at: www.dss.cahwnet.gov/getser/adpscvs.html.

American Bar Association. Commission on Legal Problems of the Elderly. Retrieved online at: www.elderabuselaw.com.

American Health Care Association. (1999). Facts and Trends. *The Nursing Facility Sourcebook, 5.*

American Public Welfare Association of State Units on Aging. *A Comprehensive Analysis of State Policy and Practice Related to Elder Abuse.* Washington, D.C. Retrieved online at: http://www.ojp.usdoj.gov/ovc/ncvrw/1996/i.

Armstrong, K.A., Kenen, R., & Samost, L. (1991). Barriers to family planning services among patients in drug treatment programs. *Family Planning Perspectives.* 23, pp. 264-271.

Bagshaw, Margaret & Adams, Mary. (1995). Nursing Home Nurses' Attitudes, Empathy, and Ideologic Orientation. *International Journal of Aging and Human Development, 22,* pp. 235-246.

Baldwin, Lewis V.(1994). *There is a Balm in Gilead: The Cultural Roots of Martin Luther King Jr.,* 224.

Berens, Michel J. (1999, May & June). Beyond the Obvious Scrutiny at America's Nursing Homes. *Chicago Tribune.*

Block, Rachel. (1999). Deputy Director of HCFA's Center for Medicaid, Testimony before the Senate Special Committee on Aging.

Bogdan, R.C., & Bilken, S.K. (1982). *Qualitative Research for Education: An Introduction to Theory Methods* (3rd ed.). Boston: Allyn & Bacon, Inc.

Boros, John. (1999). Service Employee International Union Local 250. *Nurseweek.*

Byers, Bryan & Hendricks, James E. (1993). *Adult Protective Services: Research and Practice.* Springfield, Illinois.

Bourget, Beverly. (1998). *Taking Action on Elder Abuse.* Sudbury Elder Abuse Committee, Sudbury, Ontario, Canada. Retrieved online at: http://www.cyberbeach.net/~seac/eldinst.htm.

Bourget, Beverly (1998). *Elder Abuse in Institutions.* Social Planning Council Sudbury Region. Retrieved online at: http://www.cyberbeach.net/~seac/eldinst.htm.

Bowker, Lee H. (1982). *Humanizing Institutions for the Aged.* Lexington, MA: Lexington books.

Burger, Sarah & Holder, Elma. (2000, July). *Widespread Substandard Staffing in America's Nursing Homes Needs Immediate Action.* Retrieved online at: http://www.nccnhr.org.

California State Department of Health and Human Services. Licensing and Certification Division. State Citations Issued as follows:

State Citation Issued to Nursing Home in Pleasant Hill. 2 Jun. 1999.

State Citation Issued to Nursing Home in Hayward. 12 Jul. 1999.

State Citation Issued to Nursing Home in Menlo Park   2 Sept.1999.

State Citation Issued to Nursing Home in Castro Valley 6 Aug. 1999.

State Citation Issued to Nursing Home in Walnut Creek 3 May. 1999.

State Citation Issued to Nursing Home in Alameda   27 Oct. 1999.

State Citation Issued to Nursing Home in San Jose   7 May. 1999.

State Citation Issued to Nursing Home in Oakland   24 Jun. 1999.

State Citation Issued to Nursing Home in Hayward   26 Jan. 1999.

State Citation Issued to Nursing Home in San Jose   21 Dec. 1999.

State Citation Issued to Nursing Home in Livermore   26 Jul. 1999.

Campbell, Margaret E. (1971). Study of the Attitudes of Nursing Personnel toward the Geriatric Patient. *Nursing Research, 20*, pp. 147-151.

Capezuti, E. (1997). Reporting Elder Mistreatment. *Journal of Gerontology Nursing, 23,* (7), pp. 24-32.

CBS Health Watch. (2001). One in Three U.S. Nursing Homes Cited for Abuse. Retrieved online at: http://cbshealthwatch.medscape.com/cx/viewarticle/404023.

Cheek, Julianne. (1996). Taking a View: Qualitative Research as Representation. *Qualitative Health Research, Vol.6.* Issue 4, p 492, 14p.

Cherry, R.L. (1993). Community Presence and Nursing Home Quality of Care: The Ombudsman as a Complementary Role. *Health and Social Behavior, 34,* pp. 336-345.

Colin, M. (1995). Silent Suffering: A Case Study of Elder Abuse and Neglect. *Journal of American Geriatric Society, 43,* (11), pp. 1303-1308.

Creswell, John, W. (1994). *Qualitative and Quantitative Approaches.* Thousand Oaks, London, and New Delhi: Sage Publications, Inc.

Denzin, N.K., & Lincoln, Y.S. (1994). Handbook of Qualitative Research. London: Sage Publications.

Department of Aging. Retrieved online at: http://www.oaktrees.org/elder/report.shtml.

Department of Health and Human Services. (1999). Annual Inspections of Nursing Homes. Retrieved online at: http://www.hhs.gov/news.

Doty, Pamela & Sullivan, Ellen W. (1983). Community Involvement in Combating Abuse, Neglect, and Maltreatment in Nursing Homes. *Milbank Memorial Fund Quarterly/ Health and Society, 61*, pp. 222-256.

Elder Web: California Law. Retrieved online at:
http://www.elderweb.com/region/ca/law.htm.

Elder Law FAX: Study Blasts California Nursing Homes. Retrieved online at: http://www.tn-elderlaw.com/prior/989817.html.

Elwell, Frank. (1981). *Old-Age Institutions: A Study in Social Stress.* Unpublished doctoral dissertation. Albany: Department of Sociology, State University of New York.

Ehrlich, P & Anetzberger, G. (1991). Survey of state public health departments on procedures for reporting elder abuse. *Public Health Reports*, Vol. 106, Issue 2, pp. 151-154.

Feder, M. Judith & Scanlon, William. (1980) Regulating the Bed Supply in Nursing Homes. *Milbank Memorial Fund Quarterly*, *58*, pp. 54-87.

Finkelhor, David. (1984). Common Features of Family Abuse. Beverly Hills: *Sage Publications,* pp. 17-28.

Fleishman, Rachel & Ronen, Revital. (1986). *Quality of Care and Maltreatment in the Institutions of the Elderly.* Jerusalem: Paper presented at an International Workshop on Stress, Conflict, and Abuse in the Aging Family.

Flexner, W.A., Littlefield, J. E., & Mc Laughlin, C.P. (1977). Discovering what the health consumer really wants. *Health Care Management Review*. 1, pp. 43-49.

Forrest, Harris Dr., (1993). *Ministry of Social Crisis.* 86

Frankel, Richard, M. & Devers, Kelly. (2000a). Qualitative Research: A Consumer's Guide. *Education for Health: Change in Learning and Practice, Vol. 13*. Issue 1, p 113, 11p.

Frankel, Richard, M. & Devers, Kelly. (2000b). Study Design in Qualitative Research: Developing Research Questions and Assessing Research Needs. *Education for Health*, 13, pp. 113-123.

Fredriksen, H. (1989). Adult Protective Services: Changes with the Introduction of Mandatory Reporting. *Journal of Elder Abuse and Neglect, 1,* pp. 59-70.

Friedman, Lisa. June 9, 2000. Rampant abuse at nursing homes Study finds 1 in 3 in Bay Area abused. *Oakland Tribune.*

Frolik, Lawrence & Kaplan, Richard. (1995). *Elder Law in a Nutshell.* Saint Paul Minnesota. West Publishing Co.

Grinfeld, Michael J. (2000). Nursing Home Persist as Gerontology's Greatest Challenge. *Geriatric Times, Vol. 1*, May/June, Issue 1.

Handschu, Susan S. (1973). Profile of the Nurse's Aide. *Gerontologist, 13,* pp. 315-317.

Hare, Jan & Pratt, Clara C. (1986). *Burnout: Differences between Professional and Paraprofessional Nursing Staff in Acute and Long Term Facilities.* Chicago: Paper presented to Gerontological Society of America.

Hegland, Anne. (1990). Nip Patient Abuse in the Bud: Aides Tackle Conflict Resolution. *Contemporary Long-Term Care, 64,* pp. 113-115.

Health Care Financing Administration (HFCA). *Medicare Enrollment Trends from 1966-1998.* Retrieved online at: http://www.hcfa.gov/stats/enrltrnd.htm.

Health Care Financing Administration (HFCA). *Nursing Home Care Expenditures and Average Annual Percent Change by Source of Funds Selected Calendar Years from 1970-2008.* Retrieved online at: http://www.hfca.gov/stats/enrltrnd.htm.

Health Care Financing Administration (HFCA). *Data about Individual Nursing Homes.* Retrieved online at: http://www.medicare.gov/nursing/home.asp. *Philadelphia: CARIE,* p.33.

Health Care Financing Administration (HFCA). *Study of Private Accreditation (Deeming) of Nursing Homes, Regulatory and Non-Regulatory Initiatives and Effectiveness of the Survey and Certification System.* Retrieved online at: http://www.hfca.gov/stats/enrltrnd.htm.

Heine, Christine A. (1986). Burnout Among Nursing Home Personnel. *Journal of Gerontological Nursing,* 12, pp. 14-18.

House of Government Reform Committee. *Report on Nursing Home Conditions in the San Francisco Bay Area,* 8 June 2000.

Howsden, Jackie L. (1981). *The Social Organization of the Nursing Home.* Lanham, MD: University Press of America.

Hudson, B., Soffer, B. & Menio, D. (1991). Ensuring an Abuse Free Environment. Infolink: Elder Abuse Legislation. *National Center for Victims of Crime.* Retrieved online at: http://www.nvc.org/infolink/into62.htm.

Institute of Medicine. (1986). Improving the Quality of Care in Nursing Homes. *National Academy Press.* Washington, D.C.

Jawanza, Kunjufu. (2003). African-American Images. *Black Economics,* 2nd ed.

Jones, J. (1997). Elder Abuse and Neglect: Understanding the Causes and Potential Risk Factors. *American Journal of Emergency Medicine, 15,* (6), pp. 579-583.

Jones, J. Walker, G. & Krohmer, J. (1995) To Report of Not to Report: Emergency Services Response to Elder. *Pre-hospital Hospital Disaster Med, 10,* pp 96-100.

Jones, Roger. (1995). Why Do Qualitative Research? *British Medical Journal*, Vol.311, Issue 6996, p2, 2/3p.

Kayser-Jones, Jeanie. (1981). Old, Alone, and Neglected: Care of the Aged in Scotland and the United States. Berkeley: *University of California Press.*

Kleinschmidt, K.C. (1997). Elder Abuse. *American Emergency Medicine, 30,* (4), pp. 463-472.

Kosberg, Jordan I. (1974). Making Institutions Accountable: Research and Policy Issues. *Gerontologist, 14,* pp. 510-516.

Lawton, Powell M. (1980). *Environment and Aging.* Monterey, Ca.: Brooks/Cole.

Lee, Yong S. (1984). Nursing Homes and Quality of Health Care: The First Year Result of an Outcome-Oriented Survey. *Journal of Health and Human Resources Administration, 7,* pp. 32-60.

Lieberman, A., & Tobin, Sheldon S. (1983). *The Experience of Old Age: Stress, Coping, and Survival.* New York: Basic Books.

Lincoln, Y.S., Guba, E.G. (1985). *Naturalistic Inquiry.* Beverly Hills, CA: Sage Publications.

Lofland, J., & Lofland, L.H. (1984). *Analyzing Social Settings.* Belmont, CA: Wadsworth Publishing Company, Inc.

McQueen, Anjetta. (2001). Congressional Report Says Nursing Home Abuse Rising. Associated Press: Retrieved online at: http://www.post-gazette.com/headlines/20010731nursingnat3p3.asp

Madey, D.L. (9182). Some Benefits of Integrating Qualitative and Quantitative Methods in Program Evaluations. *Educational Evaluation and Policy Analysis, 4.* pp. 223-235.

Mallis, R.M., & Lansing, D. (1986). Using focus groups to plan worksite nutrition programs. *Journal of Nutrition Education.* 18, pp. 532-534.

Marshall, C., & Rossman, G.B. (1999). *Designing Qualitative Research* (3rd ed.). Thousand Oaks, CA: Sage Publications, Inc.

Marshall, C., & Rossman, G.B. (1989). *Designing Qualitative Research.* Newbury Park, CA: Sage Publications, Inc.

Medicare and Medicaid Programs. Retrieved online at: http://www.medicare.gov.

Miles, M.B., & Huberman, A.M. (9184). *Qualitative Data Analysis: A Sourcebook of New Methods.* Beverly Hills, CA: Sage Publications, Inc.

Monk, Abraham, & Kaye, Lenard W. & Litwin, Howard. (1984). *Resolving Grievances in the Nursing Home: A Study of the Ombudsman Program.* New York: Columbia University Press.

Moos, Rudolf H. (1981). Environmental Choice and Control in Community Care Settings for Older People. *Journal of Applied Social Psychology, 11,* pp. 23-43.

National Center on Elder Abuse (NCEA). *Elder Abuse Informational Services.* Washington, D.C. Retrieved online at:

http://www.gwjapan.com/ncea/research/index.html.

Nakamura, C. W. (1987). *Innovative programmatic thrusts to teach non-traditional audiences in extension home economics.* Kahului, Hawaii: Maui County Extension Service.

National Center on Elder Abuse (NCEA). *Elder Abuse Informational Services no.2.* Washington, D.C. Retrieved online at: NCEA@NASUA.ORG.

Nix, L.M., Pasteur, A.B., & Servance, M.A. (1988). A focus group study of sexually active black teenagers. *Adolescence.* 23, pp. 741-751.

Nurse Week. *State Mandates Raise for Nursing, 13,* (15), p 2. 17 Jul. 2000.

Office of Inspector General, Department of Health and Human Services. *Resident Abuse in Nursing Homes: Respondent Perceptions of Issues.* 1 Jan. 1990.

Patton, M.Q. (1990). *Qualitative Evaluation and Research Methods.* Newbury Park, CA: Sage Publications, Inc.

Penner, Louis A., Luderria, Krista & Mead, Gayle. (1984). Staff Attitudes: Image or Reality? *Journal of Gerontological Nursing, 10,* pp. 110-117.

Pepper, Claude. (1980). Elder Abuse. Joint Hearing before the Special Committee on Aging, United States Senate, Select Committee on Aging, and the U.S. House of Representatives.

Personick, Martin. (1990). Nursing Home Aides Experience Increase in Serious Injuries. *Monthly Labor Review, 133*, (2), pp. 30-37.

Peterson, R.L., & Migler, J. R. (1987). Adjusting post-secondary agriculture curriculum to promote educational access: *An experiment.* St. Paul: University of Minnesota, Department of Vocational and Technical Education.

Pillemer, Karl. (1988). Maltreatment of Patients in Nursing Homes: Overview and Research Agenda. *Journal of Health and Social Behavior, 29*, (3), pp. 227-238.

Pillemer, Karl & Bachman-Prehn. (1991). Helping and Hurting: Predictors of Maltreatment of Patients in Nursing Homes. *Research on Aging, 13* (1), pp. 74-95.

Pillemer, Karl & Finkelhor, David. (1988). The Prevalence of Elder Abuse: Finding from a Random Survey. *Gerontologist, 28,* pp. 51-57.

Pillemer, Karl & Moore, D. W. (1990). Highlights from a Study of Abuse of Patients in Nursing Homes. *Journal of Elder Abuse & Neglect, 2,* (1), pp. 5-30.

Pillemer, Karl & Moore, D.W. (1989). Abuse of Patients in Nursing Homes: Findings from a Survey of Staff. *Gerontologist, 29,* 3. pp. 314-320.

Pope, Catherine & Mays, Nick. (1995) Reaching the parts other methods cannot reach: An introduction to qualitative methods in health. *British Medical Journal, Vol. 311,* Issue 6996, p 42. 4p.

Pope, Catherine & Ziebland, Sue. (2000). Analyzing Qualitative Data. *British Medical Journal, Issue 7227,* pp. 114-117.

Reno, J. (2000). Elder Justice: Medical/Forensic issues concerning Institutional Abuse and neglect. Paper submitted for discussion for Elder Justice: Medical/Forensic Issues Concerning Abuse and Neglect. Washington, DC. October.

Rikard, G.L., & Beacham, B. (1992). A vision for innovation in preservice teaching: The evaluation of a model program, *Action in Teacher Education*. 14, pp. 35-41.

Rosenblatt, Robert. *Problems in Nursing Homes Detailed*. Los Angeles Times. 28 July 1998. Retrieved online at: http://www.cannurses.org/can/news/ia/2898.html.

Ruppe, David. (2001). *Nursing Home Abuse*: Retrieved online at:

http://abcnews.go.com/sections/us/dailynews/nursinghomes_elderlyabuse_0107230.html

Schatzman, L. & Strauss, A. (1973). *Field Research: Strategies for a Natural Sociology*. Englewood Cliffs, NJ: Prentice Hall.

Senate Special Committee on Aging. Testimony Charlene Harrington, Professor at San Francisco University. 28 Jul. 1998.

Senate Special Committee on Aging. Testimony Rachel Block, Deputy Director of HCFA's Center for Medicaid. 30 Jun. 1999.

Senior-Site. (1990). Nursing Home Abuses. Retrieved from online at: http://senior-site.com/nursing/abuses.html.

Service Employee. (1980). *Working Together to Improve Conditions in Nursing Homes, 40,* (3), p 9. Providence, RI.

Sherman, E. & Reid, W.J., (Eds.). (1994). *Qualitative Research in Social Work.* New York: Columbia University Press.

Smith, Archie Jr. (1982). *The Relational Self.* , 23.

Smith, Joel. (2001). Nursing Home Abuse. Retrieved online at: http://www.joelsmithlaw.com/nursing.htm.

Smith, Kelly Miller Sr. (1983). *Religion as a Force in Black America.,* 201.

Snow, J.M., (Ed.). (1989). *Abuse of People: A Manual for Health Care Facilities in Newfoundland and Labrador*, St. John's, Newfoundland: Newfoundland Hospital and Nursing Home Association, p.31.

Stannard, Charles. (1973). Old Folks and Dirty Work: The Social Conditions for Patient Abuse in a Nursing Home. *Social Problems, 20,* pp. 329-342.

Steckler, A., Eng, E., & Goodman, R. M. (1991-92). Integrating qualitative and quantitative evaluation methods. *Hygie.* 10, pp. 16-20.

Strauss, A., & Corbin, J. (Eds.). (1997). Grounded Theory in Practice. Thousand Oaks, CA; Sage Publications, Inc.

Strauss, A., & Corbin, J. (1990). *Basic Qualitative Research: Grounded Theory, Procedures and Techniques*. Newbury Park, CA: Sage Publications, Inc.

Straus, Murray A. (1986). Domestic Violence and Homicide Antecedents. *Bulletin of the New York Academy of Medicine, 62,* pp. 446-465.

Stryker, R. (1981). *How to Reduce Turnover in Nursing Homes.* Springfield, IL: Thomas.

Tatara, Toshio. (1990). Elder Abuse in the United States: An Issue Paper. Washington, D.C.: National Aging and Resource Center on Elder Abuse.

Tatara, Toshio & Broughton, Debra. (1992). Institutional Elder Abuse: A Summary of Data Gathered from State Limits on Aging. National Aging and Resource Center on Elder Abuse.

Taylor, R.J., Thornton, M.C., and Chatters, L.M. (1987). Black America's Perceptions of the Socio-historical Role of the Church. *Journal of Black Studies, 18* (2), pp. 123-138.

Thompson, Mark.(1998). Shining a Light on Abuse. *Time, vol.152*, Issue 5, p 42, 2 p, 2 c.

Thompson, Mark. (1998). Shining a Light on Abuse. *Time, 3 August 1998;* pp. 42-43.

Todd, M. (1991). Elder Alert. A newsletter for senior concerns from the office of the attorney general. Vo. 6, No. 3, pp. 1-4.

Ullman, Steve G. (1985). The Impact of Quality on Cost in the Provision of Long-Term Care. *Inquiry, 2,* pp. 293-302.

USA Today. (2001). Report finds Nursing Home Abuse on the Rise. *Associated Press.* Retrieved online at: http://www.usatoday.com/news/healthscience/health/2001-07-30-nursing-home-abuse.htm.

U.S. Census Bureau. (1999) *Resident Population Estimates of the United States by Age and Sex (1990-1999).* 1 Oct. 1999. Retrieved online at: http://www.census.gov/population/www/projections/natproj.htm.

U.S. Census Bureau. (1996). *Resident Population of the United States: Middle Series Projections by Age and Sex (20015-2030).* 1 Mar. 1996. Retrieved online at: http://www.census.gov/population/projections/nation/detail/p2021_30.a

U.S. Congress, House Subcommittee on Human Services, Select Committee on Aging. *Elder Abuse: An Assessment of the Federal Response, 101st Cong.* 7 Jun. 1989.

U.S. Department of Justice. (1985) *Crime in the United States.* Washington, D.C.

U.S. House of Representatives. (2001). *Abuse of Residents Is a Major Problem in U.S. Nursing Homes*, Minority Staff, Special Investigations Division, Committee on Government Reform.

Wallace, Jonathan. (1999). Elder Abuse in Institutional Settings. *Nurse2.* pp1-9.

Walls, Carla T. (1992). The Role of Church and Family Support in the Lives of Older African-Americans. *Generations, Vol.16*, Issue 3, pp33-37.

Walter, Hanes Jr. (1976). *The Political Philosophy of Martin Luther King Jr.,* 44.

Waxman, Henry. (2001). House of Government Reform Committee. Congressional Hearings Committee Report on Nursing Home Abuse. 30 July, 2001

Waxman, Howard M., Carner, Erwin A., & Berkenstock, Gale. (1984). Job Turnover and Job Satisfaction among Nursing Home Aides. *Gerontologist, 24,* pp. 503-509.

Weihl, Hannah. (1981). On the Relationship between the Size of Residential Institutions and the Well-being of Residents. *Gerontologist, 21*, pp. 247-250.

Weiss, Carol H. (1995). *New Approaches to Evaluating Community Initiatives: Concepts, Methods, and Contexts.* Englewood Cliffs, N.J.: Prentice-Hall.

Special Consideration

Mr. Elton Brown
program director

Mr. Edward Jefferson
photographer

Nomi Nguyen
make-up artist

Donna Miranda
hair stylist

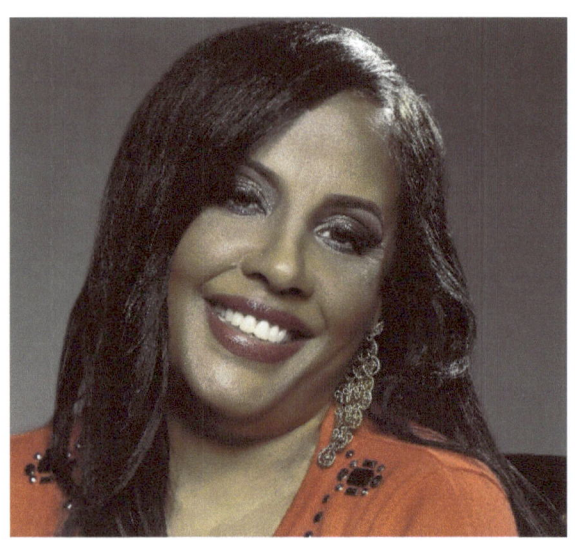

SENIORS ARE SPECIAL